THE
LIVING CLEARLY
METHOD

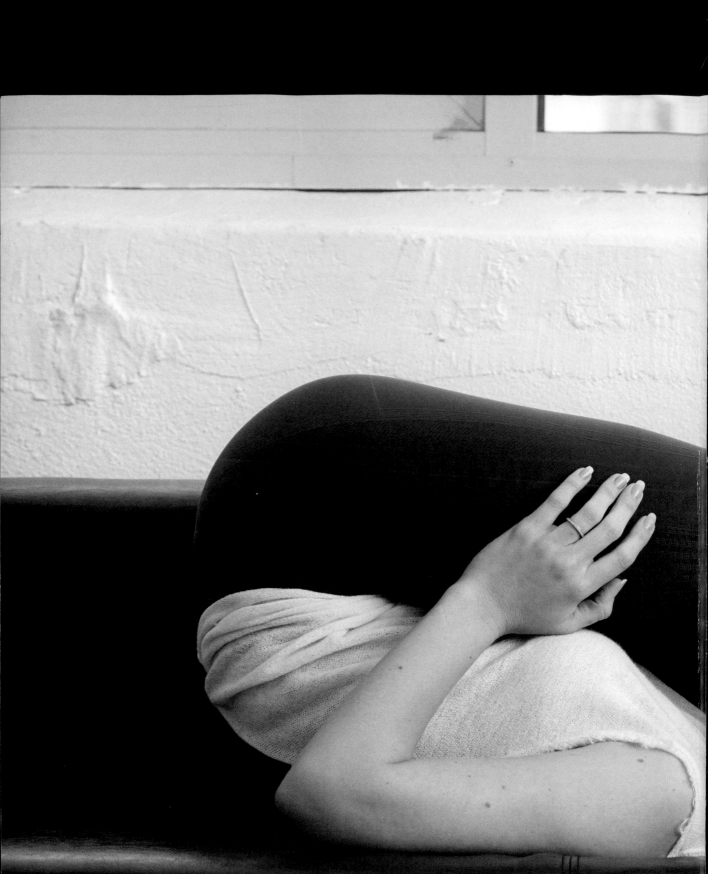

THE
LIVING CLEARLY
METHOD

5 Principles for a Fit Body,
Healthy Mind & Joyful Life

HILARIA BALDWIN

RODALE

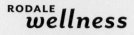

RODALE **wellness**

Live happy. Be healthy. Get inspired.

Sign up today to get exclusive access to our authors, exclusive bonuses, and the most authoritative, useful, and cutting-edge information on health, wellness, fitness, and living your life to the fullest.

Visit us online at RodaleWellness.com
Join us at RodaleWellness.com/Join

Rodale books may be purchased for business or promotional use or for special sales. For information, please write to: Special Markets Department, Rodale Inc., 733 Third Avenue, New York, NY 10017

Printed in China

Rodale Inc. makes every effort to use acid-free ♾, recycled paper ♻.

Photographs © Justin Steele: *ii–iii, v–vi, xii, 9 (bottom), 15, 18, 22, 27, 30, 37, 41, 44, 50, 52, 55-56, 59, 65, 86, 89, 94, 96, 99, 102, 108, 112, 121, 130, 135-136, 144, 148, 153, 156, 185, 197, 201, 229-230, 232, 235, 239-240, 242, 245-248*

Photographs © Rodale Inc. by Mitch Mandel/Rodale Images: *viii, 10, 34, 46–49, 62, 66, 68–74, 78–79, 81, 90-93, 101, 105–107, 116, 124–127, 143, 147, 160, 163-164, 167-168, 177, 181, 186, 191, 194, 198, 204, 206, 213, 218, 221, 243, 250*

Photographs Courtesy of Hilaria Baldwin: *5, 9 (top), 116, 140*

Book design: Rae Ann Spitzenberger
Food stylist: Lisa Homa
Prop stylist: Stephanie Hanes

Library of Congress Cataloging-in-Publication Data is on file with the publisher.

ISBN 978-1-62336-698-8 paperback

Distributed to the trade by Macmillan

2   4   6   8   10   9   7   5   3   1   paperback

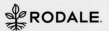

RODALE

We inspire health, healing, happiness, and love in the world.
Starting with you.

◂▾▸

This book is dedicated to *you*—
who, like me, always dreamed of a better
life, desires the perspective to know you
deserve happiness, craves the discipline
to master breathing deeply, seeks to
ground your life into a fulfilling reality,
has the playfulness to find balance in a
tumultuous world, and has the courage
to let go of negativity, even if it feels
unfamiliar. Take my hand,
let's do this together.

◂▴▸

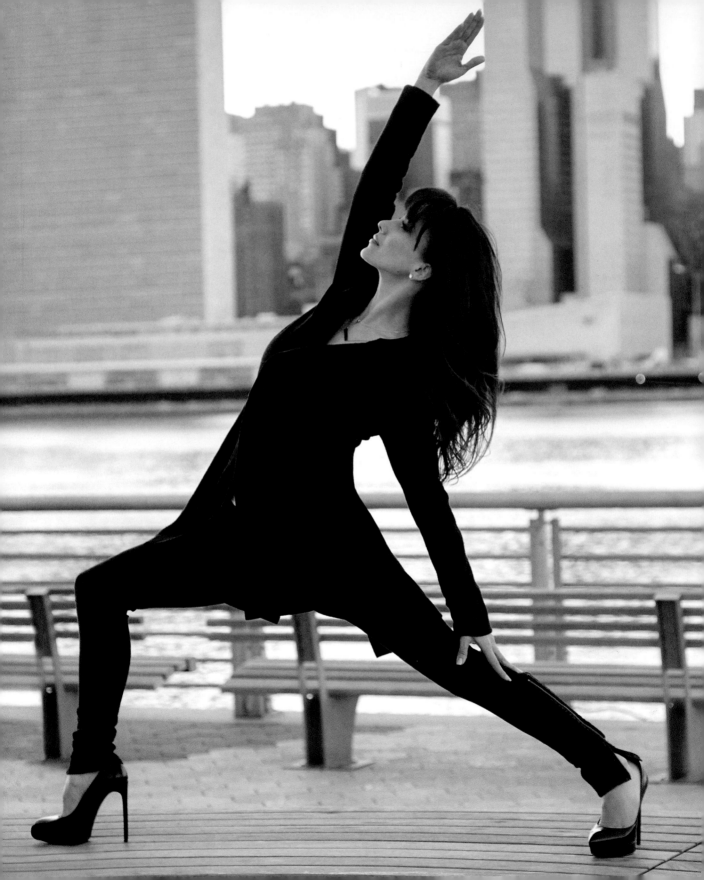

CONTENTS

Life is no brief candle to me. It is a sort of splendid torch which I have got a hold of for the moment, and I want to make it burn as brightly as possible before handing it on to future generations.

—GEORGE BERNARD SHAW

INTRODUCTION

AS A YOUNG GIRL, YEARS BEFORE I FOUND YOGA, MY GYMNASTICS COACH told me the secret to overcoming my frustration and confusion at mastering complicated moves: *There's a recipe for all of them.*

He meant that the tricky tumbling move or intricate vault exercise was actually a series of small steps. Run at the board; spring off the board; hands on vault; tuck chin; lift pelvis. Put the steps in the right sequence and the movement will unfold the way you need it to, with a clean and solid landing as the result.

It clicked. Instead of throwing myself wildly into a tricky exercise and getting banged up and angry as I failed, I followed the recipe, focusing on the first step, then the second step, then the third. This had the strangest effect: Time seemed to stretch open, I was fully inside the moment, and I felt a calm sense of control. It was like moving in slow motion and turning a blurry and confusing rush into a clear sequence of frames. To the outside world, the exercise might have looked impossibly fast and complex, but inside I was methodically and calmly executing each part of the movement and enjoying it, too.

I have thought of this lesson many times in the years since, both in my personal journey of overcoming struggles that left me feeling lost and in guiding other people on their journeys as a yoga teacher. It was an early lesson in living with awareness—being present to life as you are living it. I needed to stop going *at* life and rather be *in* life, feeling the full experience of what I was doing in each moment, instead of rushing desperately toward a goal. The gymnastics "recipes" helped me perceive the path in front of me so I could make one choice after another to get where I wanted to go. Gymnastics wasn't easy, and it was inherently effortful—but it was less complicated than I was making it.

As I've gotten older, and as my reality has become more layered and complex, I have found this to be a metaphor for making my way through life with less struggle and more meaning and joy. There are ways to slow down the rush of modern life and not feel whisked along at its mercy. There are simple recipes for perceiving the path we want to be on and making the choices to achieve our goals and dreams—be it wanting a healthier body, better relationships, more fulfilling work, or something else entirely. And there are techniques to snap out of the fog of confusion and into clarity, the place where we are present in each moment, not missing a beat, and enjoying more of it.

When I developed the Living Clearly Method as an evolution of my yoga teaching about 10 years ago, my goal was to have a system for making change that anybody could use—yoga practitioner or not. It consisted of five simple principles taught through body awareness—perspective, breathing, grounding, balance, and letting go—that could be used in any situation to combat negative patterns of behavior, clear out ways that aren't working, and make way for something new. It was, I quickly realized, a recipe for living better, my own recipe, inspired by a combination of the yoga practice I had come to love so deeply and the students who came to class.

I began testing this recipe in real life, taking it off the yoga mat and using it to come back to myself any time I was dragged off course—and soon, I began sharing these strategies with my students. Together, we discovered a formula we could use to click back into clarity when we were lost—whether in mundane complaints or serious periods of suffering. The Five Principles were a recipe for slowing down the rush and opening up the moment into a series of manageable steps—not to execute an aerial on the balance beam, but to navigate the ups and downs of everyday life.

In the years since, I've seen this relatively simple practice of yoga postures and awareness exercises help many people cut through the fog of stress and struggle and connect more authentically to themselves so they can hear what it is they truly need in order to be more happy and healthy. It helps them to stop looking outward for answers and trust what they discover from turning inward, and it helps them to find more satisfaction and meaning in their lives. Often, it brings clarity and focus to areas of health and wellness—specifically eating and working out—that have long brought confusion and disappointment.

In Living Clearly, yoga is just one facet of a brighter, more wakeful life. It is a practice that trains the body and mind, and it is also the doorway that we step through to discover a whole world of information that can help make relationships smoother, make healthy eating easier, and make working out actually work. This is the foundation that supports me every single day.

The Living Clearly Method is not a cheat to a perfect existence or a magic elixir that removes every problem from your plate. But it can, if you choose to practice it, deliver something invaluable and hard to achieve: more awareness and therefore a fuller life. Awareness is like a light inside you; it illuminates what's in the shadows so you can make better choices, and it highlights your potential so you feel calm and confident about your capacities. It lights up more of the present, helping you get more out of small moments and find satisfaction in simple things. With awareness switched on, *you* can shift the obstacles, or find peace with things you cannot change. You can choose to focus on what you already have inside and out that makes your life good, and you can light up the path that will lead you to better things ahead.

I was a dancer for many years. All performers know that the ability to drop fully into the present moment is an essential aspect to performing your very best. It is the spark that ignites all the technique and talent, catalyzing the effort you've put in, making you really shine.

My hope with the Living Clearly Method is that by giving you a simple recipe for staying present amid demands and challenges and ups and downs, it helps fan the spark of your own goals, hopes, and dreams, allowing you to experience the brightness that lies within. Perhaps that spark feels dim or hard to find right now—and I know all too well how that feels. But I also know that when you can connect inward, even the smallest ember of desire for something better can be nurtured into fire. When you commit to Living Clearly, possibility comes into focus again and change becomes within reach. As you practice each step of the recipe for connecting to yourself and staying present, something priceless is revealed. You truly get to know yourself, you discover that you are the star of your own very important story; you burn brightly, empowered from within, creating more than you ever knew you could.

It doesn't interest me what you do for a living. I want to know what you ache for and if you dare to dream of meeting your heart's longing. It doesn't interest me how old you are. I want to know if you will risk looking like a fool for love, for your dream, for the adventure of being alive. . . . It doesn't interest me where or what or with whom you have studied. I want to know what sustains you, from the inside, when all else falls away.

—ORIAH, ***THE INVITATION***

Chapter One

MY STORY

MANY PEOPLE KNOW ME AS THE WOMAN MARRIED TO ALEC BALDWIN who does yoga poses in unlikely places. But there's more to my story than that. I've worked hard to make it through the blurry parts of my life, and I've fought for the happiness that I've found.

In one of my earliest childhood memories, I'm at a playground. I was a complete monkey as a child, as comfortable climbing trees as standing on solid ground. Instead of swinging like the other kids, I shimmy across the top of the swing set, 12 feet above the ground. While this likely sent the other parents into a panic, my mother calmly calls after me, "Hilaria, are you listening to your body?" Do you trust your body with what you are doing?

Back then this was an annoying question, but I would later understand what a gift it was; I was taught to tune in to my physicality at a very young age, and this fostered my passion for movement of all kinds. My first love was ballet, which I started as a toddler (before quitting in a 3-year-old's rebellion against the too-strict teachers). Then, the free-spirited world of traditional Spanish flamenco won my heart. By age 7, I found my way into gymnastics. My small stature and agility made me a natural fit for its complex moves and rigorous training. By my early teens, I fell headlong into the world of Latin ballroom dance—equally demanding, but with tiny sequined dresses and gold lamé heels as a bonus. I loved the combination of music, costumes, and artistry. Latin ballroom was arduous yet glamorous, in a fake-tan and false-eyelashes kind of way.

My years on the competitive dance circuit gave me some incredible life skills, like focus and self-reliance. But they came at a steep price. Without realizing it, I started drifting away from the playful connection to movement I'd enjoyed as a young child and into a different and darker kind of dynamic: pushing my body to its limits and commanding it to perform through pain or fatigue. I took my instrument for granted, using my sheer mental power to override injury, smile winningly for judges and audiences, and play deaf to my aching feet, hips, and back.

By the time I got to college in New York City, I was still pushing. I took every opportunity I was given—dancing, teaching, and studying—and ignored the fact that my well-being was declining. There were times I was in so much pain I could barely walk, yet I never missed a practice or performance. Beneath my pulled-together surface, my swollen joints, strained ligaments, and ruined feet told a different story.

A long-simmering struggle with anorexia and bulimia began to hold me firmly in its grip. By the time I was 20 years old, my 5-foot-3 frame was at least 20 pounds under a healthy weight. My nails were brittle, my hair was falling out, my period was MIA, and my energy had tanked. I was miserable and desperate to feel better.

That's when I found yoga. I was hustling across the East Village to my NYU classes one day when I saw a sign for a new yoga studio. I didn't know much about the practice but heard it gave people relief from stress and physical aches and pains. Instinctively sensing that yoga might help me sustain my dance career without it destroying me in the process, I grabbed a flyer and then stared at it for a week, working up the courage to try something new—not easy for a perfectionist and competitor like me. I finally summoned up the nerve to try a basics class. Wearing baggy sweatpants and a tank top, I tiptoed to the back row with my mat.

In that first class, I discovered that yoga was the complete opposite of my dance and gymnastics training. Every posture I assumed was for my own good, not to land a high score or impress an audience. It was a revelation—and it was the first time since my mother's playground inquiry that anyone had instructed me to listen to my body. By the end of class, lying in the resting pose called Savasana, I was in tears. As a kid, I'd had such a natural connection to the part of myself that knew what would make me happy and what felt right and good, but in the swirl of competition, I'd lost touch with her. I cried because I had let her down and also because for the first time in forever, I wanted to find her again.

The owner of the studio saw potential in me and encouraged me to apprentice there and take the teacher training program. I threw myself into my studies and quickly began teaching some of the studio's large group classes.

As requests for more focused, one-on-one attention came in, I added in private classes. My sensation-based style of teaching seemed to help people struggling with all kinds of demons: eating disorders, abusive relationships, illness, obesity, addiction, anxiety, depression, and much more. We would use the yoga poses to get into the feeling of being in the body and, from that place, to find more awareness, compassion, and room for change. We explored how a physical practice could be a way into *feeling* our lives from the inside out and a key to reclaiming our power so we were not ruled by our thoughts, fears, and stories.

To maximize this, I started using special sequences of poses in my class that brought the best out of my students and helped them connect to themselves more deeply, inside the studio as well as outside it. Over time, this loose system crystallized into what I christened the Living Clearly Method. That's when I fell in love with my job. Helping others to find the seed of possibility inside themselves, even if it was just for a moment or two, lifted my heart and spirit daily.

I wish I could say that it was smooth sailing from this point on, but sometimes things have to get a whole lot worse before they get better. Even while I was helping so many others, I still didn't listen to my body. I was like the cobbler who had holes in her shoes. I spent each day teaching other people to be kinder to their bodies and to tap into the beautiful connection that yoga can create between the mind and the body, yet I was blind to how hard I was pushing myself. Like many New Yorkers who strive to make ends meet, I threw myself into teaching with relentless drive. It was my life's mission, almost a devotion, and I held myself to super-high standards. Extraordinarily long days became my reality; skipping

> We explored how a physical practice could be a way into *feeling* our lives from the inside out and a key to reclaiming our power so we were not ruled by our thoughts, fears, and stories.

meals was par for the course. Even with all the yoga I was doing, and with all the positive change that the Living Clearly Method was inspiring in others, I still hadn't found the key to tempering my go-go-go approach to life.

In 2009, one of my students approached me about opening up a yoga studio together. I jumped at the opportunity, and we spent endless hours meeting to discuss the name logo, teaching philosophy, location, and more. All this while I was still dancing, teaching dozens of yoga classes per week, running to get my cardio in, and much more. Little did I know that this amazing opportunity would get served with a very challenging lesson. It was to be the lowest point of my life.

My left hip began acting up one morning on my daily run. A lighting bolt of pain seared down my leg. I pushed through it, assuming it would eventually die down. It didn't. I'm pretty sure I have an exceptionally high tolerance for pain, but this was bigger than anything I had experienced. After a few days, the sensation progressed from discomfort to agony, and soon I couldn't get out of bed. Two doctors and bottles of painkillers later, I finally got an appointment for an MRI and a pair of crutches. The day after the MRI, I hobbled out of my apartment building with my crutches to meet some friends. I had balanced a purse on one of my shoulders, and as the apartment door closed behind me, a cold December gust blew the bag off my shoulder. As I reflexively tried to catch it, shifting to my injured leg, I heard a loud *snap* and collapsed to the pavement, landing in a pile of garbage bags. Searing pain radiated through my left hip and leg. My friends carried me back into my apartment and laid me down on the bed, where I remained, delirious from the pain, unable to eat or make it to the bathroom. Early the next morning, my doctor called with the results of the MRI. It showed that the femoral neck of my hip was barely connected to the joint. She sent an ambulance over immediately, and when I got to the hospital for emergency surgery, the surgeon deduced that the fall had actually further fractured the femoral neck, which meant that my leg bone was completely severed from my hip. It was as bad as it sounds.

Three metal pins would be holding my hip together when I woke up many hours later, writhing in pain. The doctor laid out my recovery plan: I would be wheelchair bound for 3 months. If my healing progressed, I would graduate to crutches and gradually downsize to one crutch, then to limping crutch-free. The pins would be removed about 1 year after the surgery.

As the post-op grogginess faded, the fear and claustrophobia set in. I'd lived my whole life in motion. Now, doctors were saying that if I didn't keep weight off my hip by staying in the wheelchair, they would have to fully replace my hip. The fact that I lived alone in a tiny apartment made this extraordinarily taxing, physically and mentally. Worse, we were opening our studio, Yoga Vida, in 3 weeks, and I was the antithesis of the teacher I thought I'd be on this momentous day—confined, claustrophobic, and questioning my abilities. Throughout my life, my body had performed my every command. It was my reliable and hardy tool for teaching; I was always my own best demo. Now, stripped of my physicality, I was forced to find another way to illustrate information and get my points across. In the days leading up to our opening, I would ask myself (between gripping waves of self-pity and pain): *How will I describe what it looks like when you settle into a anatomically correct Chair Pose? How will I tell them how to find a deep and expansive Warrior 1?* When opening day came, the first students filed into the studio and found me waiting at the front of the space, in my yoga pants, with my iPod cued to my favorite playlist, and sitting in a wheelchair. I was incredibly nervous.

I had to call on new powers. I had to learn to use my voice wisely and take advantage of the impact that words can have. I also discovered the power of silence, of waiting and observing the room before giving a cue. I fully grasped the power of yoga to transcend all the limitations that the mind thinks exist; yoga offers itself to every kind of body. While those early days in the wheelchair were some of the hardest of my life, they were also some of the most profound because they forced me to break out of my comfort zone and become a wiser teacher.

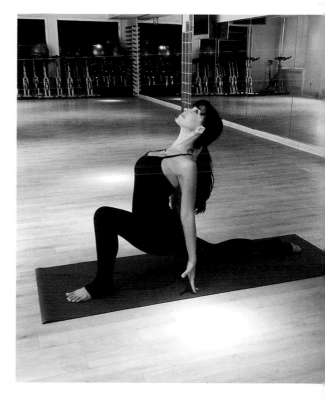

The injury was what I call a rude awakening—the moment when everything falls apart, shocking you even though in retrospect you saw it coming. This can happen to anyone—a relationship or marriage falls apart, a job goes up in flames, or you come apart at the seams under duress. When the awakening happens, it can feel like reaching rock bottom. It can also be the thing that makes you finally see.

My injury shone a glaring light on my self-sabotaging ways: My relentless drive to do more and my eating disorder were two methods I used to try to keep everything under control. I *thought* I was all about healthy living, but I was actually a bit of a tyrant to myself! I constantly demanded more of my body—perform better, work harder, sleep less, run on air and a pile of lettuce leaves. And after so much pushing, my body had screamed at me to stop through the only way it could get my attention: breaking me.

As I slowly began regaining mobility, I had a lot of time to reflect on how I was relating to my life. One day, walking slowly down the street, I had an insight that literally stopped me in my tracks: *Why can I be that whole, balanced, together person in front of an audience, but when it's just me by myself, I fall apart? Why is it important enough to be that way for other people but not important enough to be that way for myself?*

> I reclaimed that natural state of ease and freedom I'd originally had as a young girl and then lost along the way.

When that insight came, it cut through to the true feelings at my core. And what I found was not the weakness I'd feared; it was anger! I was sick of being sick and tired. I was over this self-abusive behavior. Not taking care of myself was like giving my power away. Not only had I broken my body, I had broken my relationship with myself.

This anger and passion fed my resolve to get well, once and for all. There was no quick fix to getting over my patterns, I realized. I had to learn to live my own philosophy and master the recipe of Living Clearly that I'd been teaching others. In my fervor to help as many people as possible progress in their own practice, I had completely abandoned myself.

My year of recovery turned out to be a year of waking up, in which I healed my two-decade-long eating struggle and began to treat myself right. I started to find pleasure in engaging fully with the whole process of eating, instead of checking out or avoiding it. The imbalances that had been there for much of my life returned to balance, and I looked and felt a hundred times better as a result. I began approaching exercise with a broader perspective, as well, balancing moments of high-energy physicality with greater rest and recovery.

If this phase of my life felt like the clouds parting to reveal the sun, it was because I finally found my way back into harmony with my body. I reclaimed that natural state of ease and freedom I'd originally had as a young girl and then lost along the way. I stopped letting my mind fight my body, and in place of that tension came something I now understand is absolutely essential to well-being: an acceptance of your "here and now" body as it is today and a pride in its capacity. When you cultivate that pride inside, everything external begins to shift for the better.

If you think about it, your relationship with your body is your primary relationship in life; you live 24/7 in your body. How can your relationships with other people and the world at large be healthy and positive if this fundamental one is broken and askew? Repairing my mind-body connection was like building my foundation to hold the life that I knew I wanted to have, one with a loving partner and the chance to become a mother.

But I never expected it to arrive so quickly! Just weeks after completing my year of recovery, and having stabilized my health, I felt a welcome surge of joy. One night, I headed out with two girlfriends for a meal. I was feeling celebratory; I was fit and healthy again, and my business partner and I had found a second location for our expanding yoga studio. We decided to treat ourselves to a glass of wine alfresco, as it was an unseasonably warm evening. Enjoying ourselves, my girlfriends and I chatted about everything from work to fitness to dating. Feeling very clear about what I wanted, I declared to the sky, "Universe, I'm ready to meet someone and fall in love!"

Little did I know that by a stroke of destiny my husband-to-be was sitting just two tables away, and perhaps he'd intercepted the message. My girlfriend whacked me on my leg, whispering, "Hilaria, shut up! Alec Baldwin is looking at you." I peered over to his table and saw him staring and smiling at me. I recognized him, but only barely, because I hardly ever went to the movies or watched TV. Playfully, I winked at him before turning back to our conversation. As I left the restaurant, he grabbed my hand, looked me square in the eye, and said, "Who are you? I must know you." The clarity of his intention stopped me in my tracks. I told him it was a cheesy line but took his card when he gave it to me. I assumed we would never see each other again.

A few days later, when a friend spontaneously dialed the number on the card from my phone, determined that I say yes to whatever new adventures life threw at me, our fate was sealed. Our connection was immediate and strong, yet we got to know each other in stages, very deliberately, talking intimately about what we wanted. It was the epitome of thoughtful dating and, looking back, ridiculously proper; it took 6 weeks of Alec shaking my hand after our dates before he asked permission to kiss me. As we fell in love, my husband-to-be held a vision of our shared future with absolute certainty. I listened deeply to my heart, letting it guide me past any hesitations about our different ages or lifestyles. The truth was undeniable: We clicked together. Loving Alec felt so good and so right—and we had so much fun.

I guess as much as I've discovered the art of slowness, I'm calibrated for quick. We married a little over a year after we met, with scores of our friends and relatives dancing to flamenco music at our wedding party. Our beautiful daughter, Carmen, was born the year after, and 2 years after that, we welcomed our cherished son Rafael. And our family is still growing. I wrote this book while pregnant with our third child, a little boy. My children are the lights of my life. And they have proven to be complete monkeys, like me, climbing and scampering with a natural glee. I watch and encourage every move, knowing one of the best skills I can teach them is to trust, listen to, and honor their bodies.

Alec and I have a Spanish phrase engraved on our wedding rings: *Somos un buen equipo,* which means "We are a good team." We lean on each other for help, we push each other to try harder, and we see the other's potential on those inevitable days when we forget. In this way, we can help each other stay clear and present amid the ever-changing events and circumstances of our lives. It's hard for any of us to do this alone; there is too much coming at us today, distracting us and pushing us off the path. My hope for this book is that it helps you feel part of *un buen equipo*, with me as your guide and the many other women and men who are reading it standing alongside you, as well. My work as a teacher has taught me something powerful: While we are all individuals, with unique gifts and assets that should be enjoyed and celebrated, we are also more similar and more connected to each other than we can even dream. My biggest goal in Living Clearly is that you feel this connection and know you are not in this alone.

I have road tested my techniques and fine-tuned the recipes for keeping body and mind together. Now I want to share some of what I've done with you. I invite you to take off your shoes, flex your toes, stretch your hands over your head, and step into an experience of connecting with yourself and trusting all that you discover within.

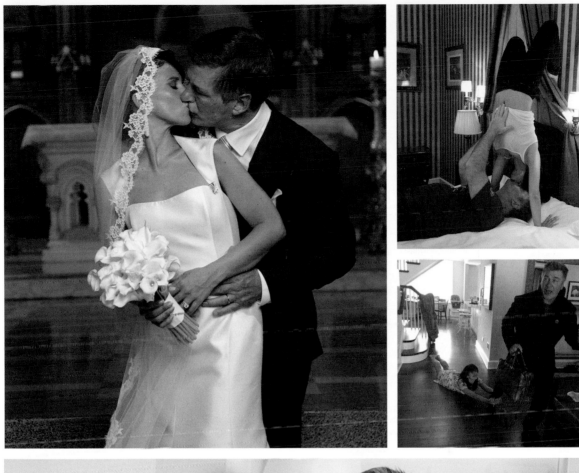

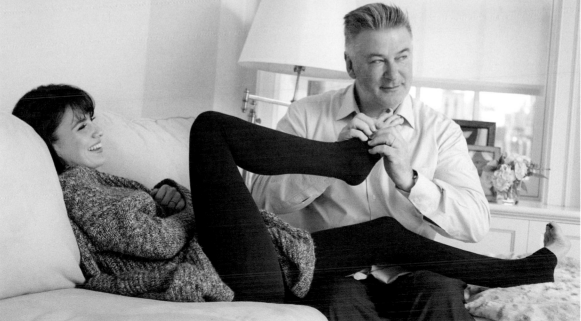

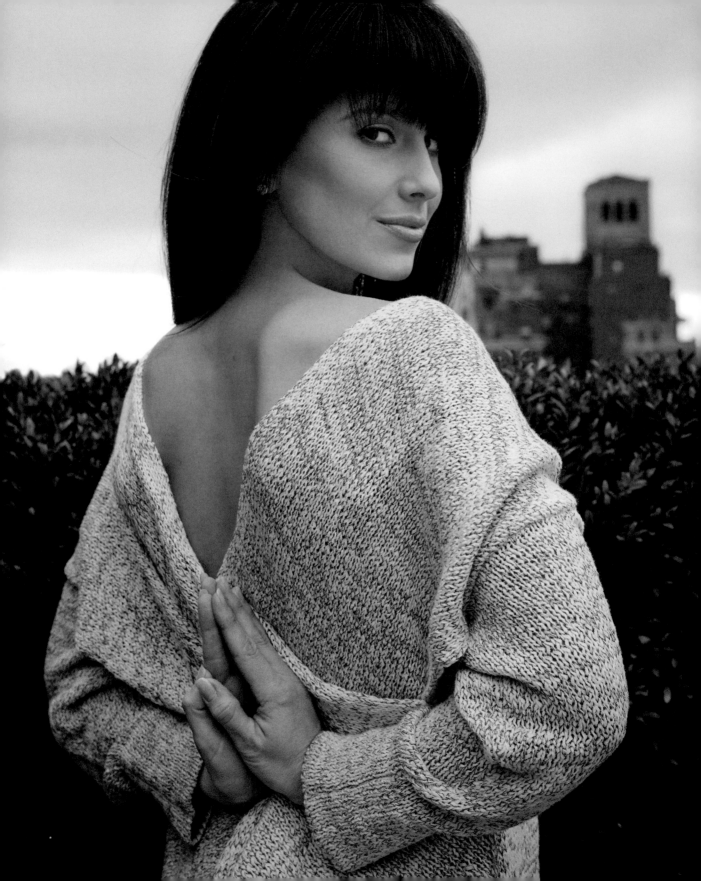

Chapter Two

THE LIVING CLEARLY METHOD:
CONNECTING THINKING AND FEELING

WHEN PEOPLE COME TO ME FOR ONE-ON-ONE YOGA SESSIONS, NO MATTER what the issues are that bring them there, one universal question always comes up: *What gets in the way of your life unfolding the way you want it to?* When we drill down to uncover the answer, we usually find that the obstacle isn't something external like a tough schedule or a busy job; it comes down to the micro-moments when they are faced with choosing between doing something supportive for themselves or doing something sabotaging, and they find themselves doing the latter.

We all do it! I know I did for years. Every day presents so many opportunities to go one way or another: to blend up a healthy smoothie or grab a packaged snack; to get up and go running or slump onto the couch; to respond calmly to a melting-down child, partner, or colleague or lose your patience. Life is a series of choices, and we often don't feel in control of the choices we make. In fact, we're often not even aware these *are* choices; our ways of acting are so habitual, they are grooved into us—they are patterns. We get ourselves in ruts that are hard to get out of, and sometimes we get stuck.

Not working out. Working out too much. Not eating enough. Eating too much. Avoiding fresh vegetables. Avoiding being alone. Giving your energy away to the wrong people. Checking out with technology. OD'ing on coffee and sugar (or much worse) even though you want to quit. These patterns can manifest in a lot of different ways, and balance can be a constant struggle.

Why don't we always choose what serves us best? My own journey out of the fog has provided me with endless opportunities to ask this and work on the answer. I never found talk therapy to be fully effective in resolving my sabotaging behaviors. My mind was such a good, A+ kind of student that I would agree with everything the therapist said about the issues that blocked me—but I'd go home and repeat the same bad choices again.

What I discovered through yoga was that none of that smart thinking would make a difference until I connected thinking with *feeling* and found my way into the situation through my living, breathing body.

We all have moments when we feel powerless to make the good choice—it's called being human—and though we can blame the situations in our lives until we're blue in the face, it actually stems from a disconnect between body and mind. This disconnect runs deep, but it can be mended. Let's look at it a little closer.

MIND AND BODY: FRIENDS OR STRANGERS?

Did you know you speak two languages? Your mind speaks a verbal language; it uses words with amazingly persuasive power. It's loud, convincing, and pretty bossy. It uses its way with words like an authority, telling you what to do, how to do it, and when to do it. The mind is also insecure, inconsistent, and can be somewhat self-destructive. The mind likes the past and the future; it uses yesterday's experiences and speculation about tomorrow to make decisions.

The body speaks a different language. It communicates through sensation and feeling and is much quieter than the mind's noisy monologue. It makes itself known through subtle messages—desires and impulses and involuntary actions like a spike of hunger in the belly or an arch and stretch of a spine that's gotten stiff. The body lives in the now; it is completely present tense. Feed me, rest me, touch me, heal me.

These two parts of ourselves need to be in good communication, working as a team. The body is a pleasure-seeker, and left to its own devices, it would have us spend our days lounging blissfully in a meadow, doing nothing but eating and sleeping. Its feelings can be extremely primal—have you ever felt your blood boiling with rage or heart spiking with fear? The mind is the more intellectual side; it helps us to actually navigate the complex world. It takes in context, consequence, and the bigger picture. At that boiling point, it's the mind that decides to relax, breathe, and calm things down. To survive and thrive, nature designed us to have a harmonious and balanced relationship between the two.

SIGNS OF A STANDOFF

When mind and body aren't communicating well, you can feel:

▸ **Stuck and confused.** You know you should be making a healthy choice but the faster or more convenient or less effortful one often wins. Breaking out of the steely grip of a craving just seems like more work. Green juice? Nah, I need the double mochaccino.

▸ **Uncomfortable or unwell.** Pushing past exhaustion or staying too sedentary takes a toll on health, looks, and self-esteem. Frustrated or disgusted, you ignore the body even more, miss the signals of illness or injury, and eventually pay a really high price.

▸ **Lost or adrift.** Living primarily in the head, you ignore your gut feelings, which exist to balance out reasoning and logic and guide you to what serves you best. The mind is a dreamer and a great storyteller. When it dominates, you spin your wheels—doubting, speculating, and projecting instead of taking action and think your way into realities that are limiting or not even true.

▸ **At war with yourself.** When your two sides are locked in combat, you are no longer working *with* your body. You're positioned against it. How could you possibly treat yourself well or feel good about who you are and what you've achieved? This can lead to self-sabotaging or self-abusive behaviors.

But in today's pressure-cooker world, we're way out of balance; the mind has gotten so overbearing that we almost can't hear the body's needs anymore. We live in the realm of the mental, pretty much all the time—thinking, processing, and obsessing while being bombarded with global news 24/7, endless to-do lists, and high-stakes strategizing about keeping our families and finances together. It's almost impossible to stay connected to our bodies' messages in the heat of the modern moment. The language of the body is not high-tech. The body is not focused on goals, ambitions, and rewards. It actually needs a slower, softer space to be heard. (Which is why you always feel more in touch with yourself on vacation.) It might tell you that you're craving simple healthy food, plenty of good sleep, daily exercise, and loving touch. But the mind orders you otherwise: There's no time to shop and cook! Self-care is indulgent! Don't stop or you will fall through the cracks! With the body pleading one way and the mind urging another, which side do we trust? There's a fundamental split in our experience, and knowing what to do and even what we *want* is confusing. Which makes daily decisions like what to eat or how to exercise such a struggle.

During my darkest points, I didn't know how to listen to myself or connect to my feelings and needs at all. And I couldn't see my own responsibility for the obstacles I faced. No wonder my life couldn't unfold the way I wanted it to. Being deaf to my body's wisdom was like driving down a mountain road with a dirty windshield and no GPS.

Worst of all, this disconnect robs you of the present moment. Consumed with stress and struggle, you often miss the simple moments that give meaning to a day—a peaceful morning alone, a smile shared with a stranger. Deprived of this, life can feel like it is passing you by more quickly than it is. This is perhaps the greatest tragedy of all.

A CLOSER LOOK AT CLARITY

How often in your life do you pause and listen—really listen—to what your body wants to do?

Do you ever tune in to your rumbling belly and ask it, What kind of hunger is this? Hunger for a hearty lunch or a power snack—or am I really just hungry for distraction because there is too much work on my plate?

Do you ever ask your tight back, What would make you feel better right now? Do you need to stretch and bend, right here by the desk, or walk around the office?

Do you notice tightness in your chest or butterflies in your stomach and ask, What would

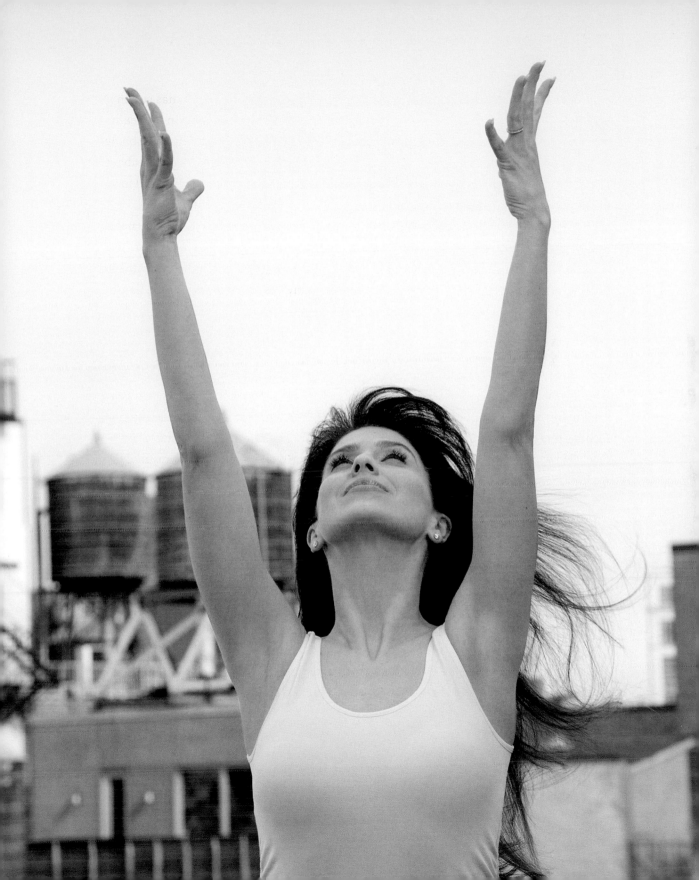

calm me right now? Running outside in the sun? Sinking my feet in the grass? Playing with the dog?

How often do you stop what you are doing and take one of those actions?

Ask people what "clarity" feels like and they might use words like *awake* or *alive*. They might say that when they have clarity, their bodies feel alert and their minds are focused or they feel sure of themselves and certain about what to do. If you think about it, it sounds like a human being operating in an uncomplicated and optimal way: balanced and whole, unhindered by doubt or confusion.

And it is, because clarity comes when the mind is connected to the body's intelligence, as nature designed it to be. In this state, the lines of communication are open between them. We're intimately aware of this intelligence when we are kids; it's what drives all our choices, because the mind's skills of analyzing and rationalizing are not yet developed. It's the part of us that doesn't really care what other people think or whether it's appropriate to ask for "more." It expresses the need of the present moment in basic terms: Give me food, water, hugs, or sleep. Or perhaps more accurately, it's about what feels good: Let me run naked with my rain boots on, paint butterfly wings on my back, and stick my face into my birthday cake!

Of course, as children, that mind-body conversation is very one-sided. It's mostly body with minimal mind—which means lots of present-moment desires and little longer-term thinking. That balance shifts as we grow and evolve, and in an ideal world, it would arrive and stay at a harmonious center point, where enlivened body intelligence communicates easily with a mind that listens.

It's vital that the mind does weigh in as we age; it's what guides us out of the childhood garden and through the complexities and nuances of life. The mind's job is to factor in the context of the current situation, consider consequences, and gather additional information from other sources. It runs all the data through its mega-computer and evaluates what action to take to safely and effectively meet the need at hand. When the lines of communication are open between body and mind, there's a partnership, a team effort: First, the body's needs are fully heard and honored; then broader considerations like personal responsibilities, other peoples' needs, and limiting circumstances are factored in, as well. When the body says it wants to jump in the ocean right now, the mind points out that you actually have a job you have to be at and that it's freezing out, and it decides that a sprint around the block will have to do.

FINDING THE WAY BACK

There is a way back. We can retrain the mind to listen to the body and encourage the body to speak more loudly so that the two sides come back into conversation.

Yogic philosophy teaches that by moving the body with deep attention and care, you can create a sensation inside that is so compelling to the mind that it turns to look inward instead of facing outward. With a big breath that fully expands the lungs and makes the mind go, "Wow, that feels different!" or through a satisfying stretch that opens a muscle group that's been tense for a long time or through the amazing sensation of raising your body heat, the mind's interest is piqued, it is drawn within. Turning inward means the thoughts and stimulation of the outer world—and of your own loop of stories, beliefs, and judgments—start to fade into the background. You can hear your inner language of sensations and feelings. This creates the state of simple, focused awareness where you can experience clarity. With mind and body equal partners, you see priorities you couldn't see before, and you are clearer on what action to take that's best for you, which makes it easier to follow through.

> We can retrain the mind to listen to the body and encourage the body to speak more loudly so that the two sides come back into conversation.

Perhaps you perceive, *I'm agitated and antsy— I really need to work out! Or, I'm feeling sad and vulnerable, so I'm going to reach out to friends and get nurtured.* By connecting thinking and feeling, you can also problem solve on your behalf in a compassionate way. You see that although you can't realistically connect with a friend tonight for much-needed comfort and solace, you can still pick up a soothing book for 5 minutes, make a warm cup of tea, or write in your journal. Working together, the mind and body always find the way.

When mind and body reunite as teammates, it is such a relief! The tug of war can end, leaving you so much more mental and emotional room to do the things that are really good for you, like taking care of your body, nurturing your family, or pursuing a dream. The struggle ceases because mind and body are finally in the same place at the same time: in the present moment. They are working in sync and harmonious, motivated by the same great goal of taking care of you in the best way possible. You become, even if just for a moment, fully present to yourself.

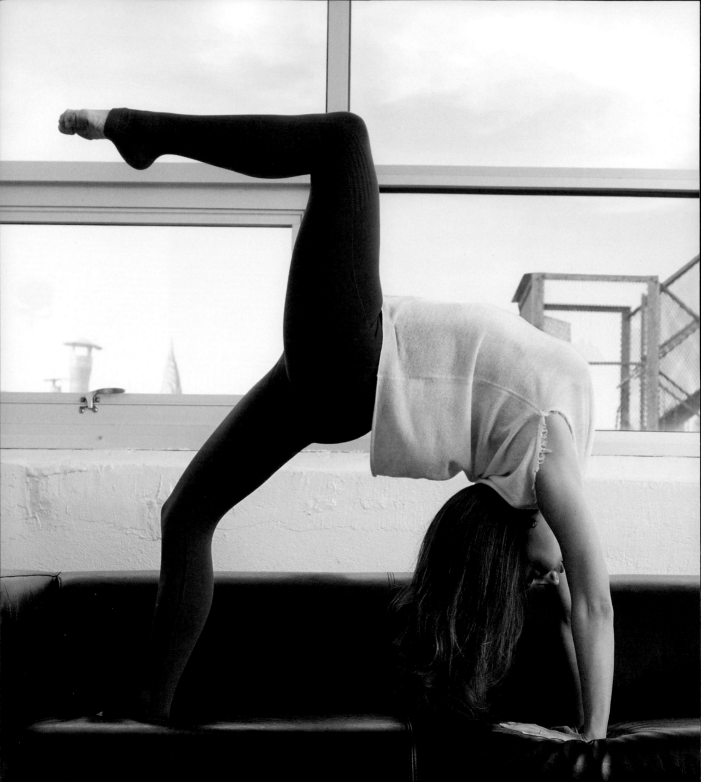

And when you return to this balanced state, you wake up the joy and pleasure of being in your body that you might not have felt for some time, the joy that often gets blocked by negative self-talk and poor self-image. Turning up the body's vital language of feeling and sensation starts to drown out those messages so you can feel that childlike joy again—the energy that makes you want to jump, run, and dance, for fun. You don't have to be a marathoner or an expert yogi to feel your muscles activated and your lungs expanding and contracting. All you need is a body and a little awareness. Simply being active, you click into the wonder of your physical form and feel its complex machinery in action. That itself is a victory.

THE LIVING CLEARLY METHOD

The Living Clearly Method starts with listening to yourself and creating a connection through yoga, but that's just the beginning. I use postures to contact the innate awareness, or inner guidance, that can get muffled or silenced in the overwhelming noise of everyday life, and amplify its voice. Then I show you how to take this connection to your outer experience, where it will guide you to make better choices in three key areas: the way you respond to life as it comes at you, the way you feed your body, and the way you move it through exercise.

This book is not designed to be read completely sitting down! You'll be invited to move, stretch, and adopt some simple yoga poses and then experience complete yoga flows. I've found this to be the fastest way to truly get the lessons. And it is an available and accessible way: We all have a body. We can start practicing right now. Your feet, hips, chest, shoulders, and back will be your tools and teachers in this process.

In Part One, you will discover the Five Principles—five simple ideas and practices that will help you relate to yourself better, to other people, and to the world at large. By bringing new awareness to the way you respond to things, they help to break patterns of stress and reactivity and to improve how you get through each day.

In Part Two, Food and Fitness, you'll learn to bring the practice to the way you take care of yourself physically. Food is one of the biggest influences on how you feel and perceive your world. Exercise is one of the quickest ways to clear the mind and energize the body. In each of these sections, I'll share how the Five Principles can transform your relationship with eating and exercising, and then I'll share the systems I use to easily and effectively make healthy food and regular exercise consistent parts of my life.

Living Clearly is not a set plan or a methodology to follow for 30 days and then drop. The goal is for the tools in this book to become things that integrate gradually and naturally into your life. There's no perfectionism allowed here! It's just about the practice, and practice means showing up without being overly attached to a goal. Practice also means consistent, routine behaviors. Keep practicing the Living Clearly Method, and over time you will know yourself better, treat yourself better, and achieve greater health and well-being as a result.

I love to read inspirational quotes as my yoga students stretch and open physically or as they prepare to rest and let go. One of the passages I've turned to over and over was written by the poet Rainer Maria Rilke and later published in the collection *Letters to a Young Poet*.

Have patience with everything unresolved in your heart and . . . try to love the questions themselves as if they were locked rooms or books written in a very foreign language. Don't search for the answers, which could not be given to you now, because you would not be able to live them. And the point is, to live everything. Live the questions now. Perhaps then, someday far in the future, you will gradually, without even noticing it, live your way into the answer.

My journey of living the questions has convinced me that even if we can't improve every part of our lives, we can become more present to them. We can become more resilient in the face of pressures and challenges; we can derive more joy from the great parts and gain wisdom from the hard parts. We can step through the confusion, turn away from distraction, learn to like ourselves more, and practice living every minute that we have.

The journey starts with a first step, bringing new awareness to how you relate to your life.

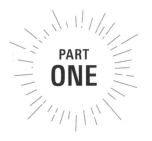

PART
ONE

THE FIVE PRINCIPLES

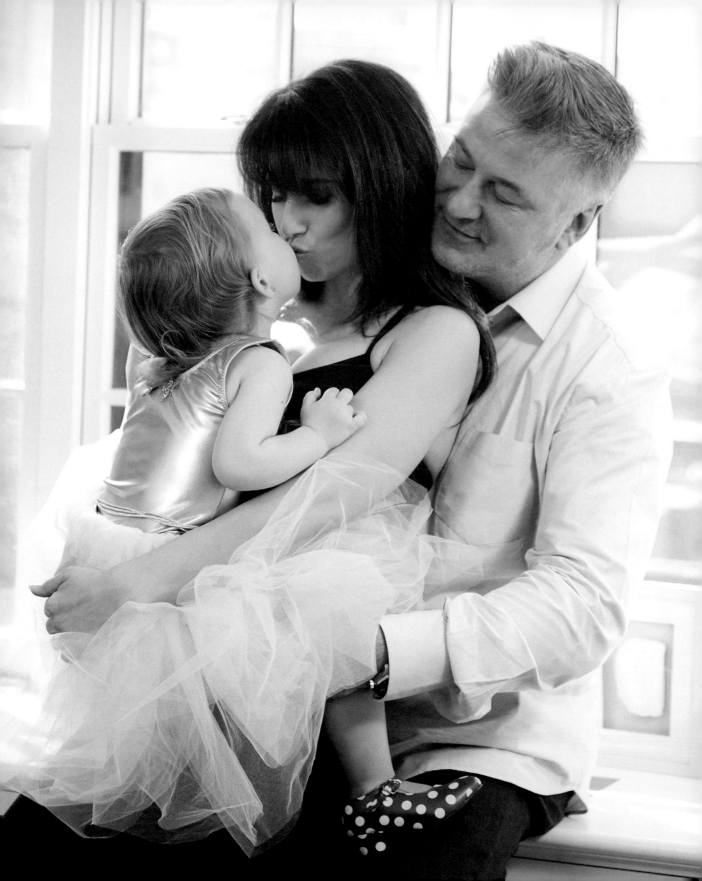

Chapter Three

RELATING CLEARLY

LIVING CLEARLY STARTS AND ENDS WITH HOW YOU RELATE TO YOUR world. Yup—it's really that simple. Your happiness, health, and vibrancy are born from how you interface with the people in your life, how you deal with the inevitable challenges that come your way, and, most essentially, how kind you are to yourself in the process. Years of wiping the fog off my own windshield, and witnessing my students do the same, has shown me that genuine clarity—and the mental, emotional, and physical vibrancy that comes with it—is totally and completely dependent on the way we *relate* to everything that comes our way, internally and externally.

But what is "relating"? It is the action component of relationship; it's the fire, the juice, the chemical combustion that happens when two separate entities face off. In your own life, these entities could be you and your current love interest, you and your boss, or you and a luscious piece of chocolate cake. When it comes to relating, the other entity doesn't have to be a living, breathing human being. It can be a thing, a concept, a belief structure, or a situation. You relate just as much to the reflection you see in the mirror each morning or the traffic you're stuck in, the job you're stuck in, or the relationship you're stuck in as you do to your kids or your friends. And relating also applies to our habits. How do you relate to tobacco, alcohol, TV, sex, chocolate? Are you in a healthy relationship with the things that tempt you and pull you away from what you know is really good for you?

Most of the relating we do is unconscious. We sleepwalk through our days, allowing ourselves to get dragged around by our desires and emotions like a puppy on a leash. Our reactions are automatic and habitual: We see the chocolate cake, and we reach for it. Stuck in the traffic jam, we steam, pout, or fret. Our spouse yells at us, and we yell back. We're like a Ping-Pong ball being swatted from one side of the table to the other, again and again, over the same net. It's easy to forget that we don't have to do things the same way, that we don't have to remain a prisoner of reactivity. There is always a new path or better choice we can make.

> It's so exciting to realize that in every moment of every day we have the option to shift how we relate to whatever is showing up for us right here, right now.

It's so exciting to realize that in every moment of every day we have the option to shift how we relate to whatever is showing up for us right here, right now. If the coffee you ordered arrives lukewarm or your love connection loses its spark or you get fired, insulted, or shoved—*you* decide how you're going to relate to the situation. Whether you're running late for a ridiculously important meeting, struggling to relocate your butt from the couch to your spin class, or frantically excavating your closet in hopes of nailing an outfit for a promising date, *you* choose how you're going to deal with the situation. And while most of the relating we do is centered around daily conflicts or challenges, in the course of a lifetime, we'll also be asked to relate to circumstances with much higher stakes, such as mourning the loss of a loved one, managing a difficult diagnosis, or facing depression, addiction, or anxiety. The ways in which we relate to something or someone are massive *and* tiny; they rock the foundation of who we are, and they bounce off the surface leaving barely a dent.

I could fill this book with examples of how human beings are asked to relate to heartbreak, frustrations, conflict, and disappointments. The examples are endless and universal; nobody escapes the hard stuff. In fact, you've likely experienced many of the situations I've listed above, probably this week or today, and it's 100 percent guaranteed that you'll experience zillions more, in predictable and totally surprising manifestations. And as they've done in the past, these challenging situations will stir up some pretty real feelings: anger (maybe even rage), hopelessness, despair, confusion. Maybe you see that the way you relate to your world is being influenced by laziness, addiction, or some other bad habit—powerful forces that can be difficult to fight. Thankfully, you can begin to point yourself in a new direction—to break a pattern and liberate yourself from the sticky web of reactivity—by simply creating enough space to choose a softer, kinder, more honest approach to whatever or whomever you're facing.

Create space. That sounds great. But how do regular people with regular responsibilities, regular insecurities, and the usual temptations go about creating some metaphorical space that will change how they relate to a moody spouse or tantrum-prone toddler or the 10 pounds they want to lose? The answer is deceptively simple: Connect the mind and body to gain clarity. I have used yoga to really drive myself toward this goal. The stretching, strengthening, and balancing that you do in the average yoga class is a single aspect of a complex philosophical system that's really, really old and carries some timeless wisdom. Physical postures, or asanas, are one of the eight limbs or paths that makes up the wider yogic universe. If you were to study yoga in its entirety, you'd come across intricate and esoteric texts about achieving a calm mind and a peaceful heart, hundreds of techniques and practices for preparing the body to quiet the mind through meditation, lots of hard-to-pronounce Sanskrit words (the ancient language of the practice), and countless photos of bendy men and women twisted into impossibly pretzel-like poses. It can all be a bit intimidating, especially to the new practitioner.

What I have felt on my own yoga mat and have witnessed as a teacher to thousands of New York yogis, of all shapes and sizes, of all ages and fitness levels, is that yoga is an incredibly generous system for health and well-being. The philosophical teachings of yoga are open to interpretation and adaptation. Like the yoga master who easily wraps his legs around his head, they can be bent to fit your own life.

PERSPECTIVE, BREATHING, GROUNDING, BALANCE, AND LETTING GO

The Five Principles of Living Clearly were born from the understanding that we each come in with a deep knowing that naturally guides us to a strong and healthy body, calm mind, and happy heart, but through life's challenges and traumas, we lose that understanding, slipping further and further away from the true essence of who we are.

Each principle starts and ends with *attention, intention,* and *conscious action.* You must first see what is holding you back (attention), acknowledge that you want to change it (intention), and then take a teeny tiny step toward that change (action). This is far from easy, but that one small step sends a signal to your mind that you're serious about doing something better for yourself. Then the next step becomes a little easier, and the one after that even easier. Before you know it, bam! You've activated a new way of being.

Each of the Five Principles is a tool you can use to change the way you relate to your world: how angry you get, how much joy you feel. These tools are free and available to everyone at every moment, and the opportunities to use them are endless. I lean on them constantly to make quick choices about how to deal with situations and emotions: how to deal with overzealous paparazzi (befriend them), how to work through an argument with my husband (kiss him—yup, midfight), or how to juggle a sleepless toddler with a hungry infant (bring them all into bed with me).

Luckily, mastering the principles does not require studying hard-to-understand texts or sitting through lengthy lectures. The gateway to each principle is through a specific area of the physical body, and each one can be practiced by moving into simple yoga poses. Yoga postures give the body an opportunity to experience the felt sense of the Five Principles, which helps the mind integrate the teachings held within each.

For example, if you're feeling anxious and it seems as if you're floating off the ground with worry and concern, you could say to yourself: *I want to be more grounded in this moment; I want to trust that everything is going to be okay.* But if your body can't recall what, exactly, it feels like to be grounded, your mind will spin around fuzzy mental constructs, grasping for something. The *felt experience* of the body helps to embed the sensation of each principle into your being.

Each of the yoga poses in this chapter is your path into the wisdom of the principle. When you move your body into a specific posture, one that has been assumed by millions

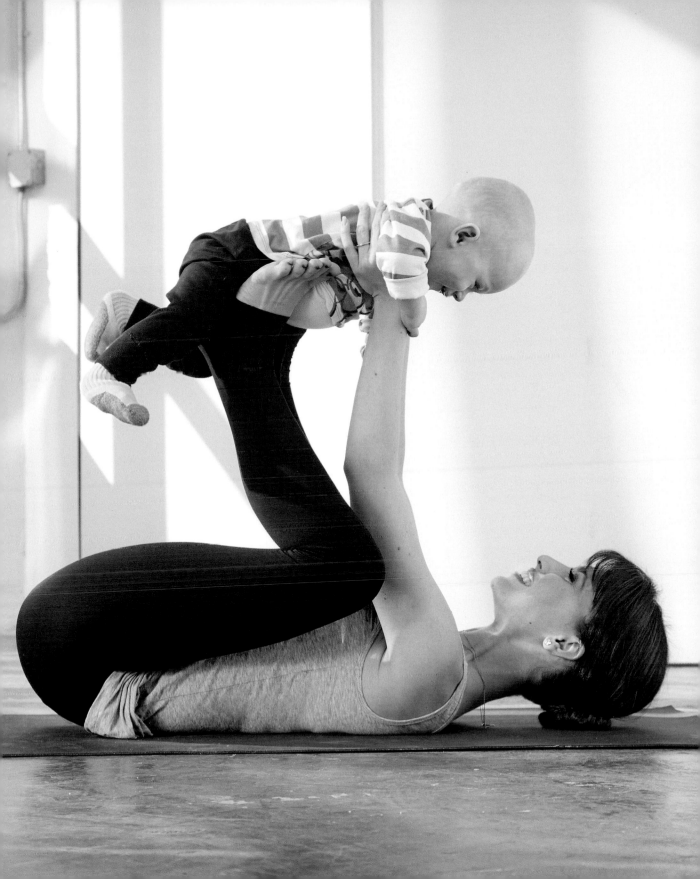

HOW TO USE THE YOGA POSES AND FLOWS

Yoga's benefits are diverse and far-reaching. It conditions every part of the body in incredibly efficient ways. It will strengthen some body parts while stretching others, sometimes in a single pose. This promotes balance in the body and a more harmonious and integrated state of mind. It promotes mobility by enhancing strength and flexibility and supporting healthy joint function. The result is that yoga powerfully counterbalances the soreness and stiffness that comes from sedentary modern lifestyles. It also makes any other activity you do—from gardening to golf—come easier and feel better.

By stimulating the internal organs and the meridians, the invisible pathways of energy that flow throughout a human being, yoga helps the body do its essential jobs of digesting, healing, and rebuilding and helps the brain to think more clearly. It stimulates your endocrine system to release feel-good chemicals like oxytocin, and a challenging practice might also release endorphins. By promoting better circulation, it helps your body release physical toxins; by calming the nervous system, it helps toxic thoughts dissolve, as well. Yoga slowly and safely softens the armor of tight, stressed muscles that almost all of us wear daily. As more space is created in the body, the consequence is almost always that we feel more space in our lives.

As you read each chapter, experiment with the individual poses and exercises scattered throughout as well as with the yoga sequences at the end of each principle. It's best to wear comfortable clothes while moving through the poses (though my Instagram yoga-pose-of-the-day photos have proven you can do more than a few poses in stilettos, a cocktail dress, or winter parka). And though any flat surface will work, it's nice to practice on a yoga mat so you don't slide around. The most important thing is that you play with these movements—at home, at work, or while waiting on line at the bank. In Chapter Ten, you'll read more about using yoga as part of your workout program. With repetition, you'll find you don't need to look at the book as closely and can get into the experience more deeply.

Yoga's real gift is the way it challenges the mind to stay present and not wander and invites you to use every part of yourself to the best of your ability. I always encourage my students to give it their all, not by applying brute force but by applying full intention and effort—to hold a pose longer, to try a balance again and again, or to sink deeply into the floor in Savasana and truly let go. I want them to not shy away from sensation, and I encourage you to do the same with the poses and sequences throughout the book. By the end of a good yoga session, you should feel "used up" in a good way. From top to toe and inside and out, you should feel worked and awakened. The armor melts through the heat of breathing and movement and suddenly there is an opening. It is a contented exhaustion. Give each moment your all, and on the other side of it, you will feel a tremendous release.

of yogis before you, you are tapping into a system that actually enmeshes the way of the principle it represents into your being. Instead of filing the principles away in some dusty folder in the back of your mind, you begin to know them in your muscles, bones, and cells; they become part of you.

I chose yoga as a way into experiencing the theoretical content of the Five Principles because it is a system of movement and philosophy of well-being that I trust. It is often described as the union between body and mind, connected by the breath. Sometimes the aesthetic of a lean, toned yoga body is what draws a person to trying yoga, and he or she discovers mindfulness as a side effect. Other times, mindfulness—and the promise of stress relief and relaxation—is the allure and fitness is the side effect. In my method, both these things go hand in hand. Fitness and mindfulness are the double outcome of the practice; you practice mindfulness in every movement, and your movements get more effective and more transforming because of that connected state.

Take comfort in the fact that you already know how to do this. Whether you know it or not, you've been in a conversation with your body for your entire life. From the moment you were born, your body has been talking to you, telling you exactly what it needs, sometimes just taking what it wants. You stretch when you need to wake up and start the day, your stomach rumbles when it is hungry, and you clench your fists or your jaw and your breath shortens when you're angry. Some of these actions are involuntary, but many can be controlled consciously. In fact, you are actually sitting at the control panel of the vessel that is your body. You have the power to decide how you want to feel by paying attention to what your body is telling you and choosing a different or better response (what would happen if you loosened your jaw and breathed deeply during a conflict with your spouse?). Practicing yoga postures and breathing techniques of the Five Principles is a way to train your body to create more space between anger and reactivity, between frustration and blaming, which leads to fewer angry and frustrated moments and more laughter and joy. And as you put the principles into practice in your life, they become reliable tools to assist you through any challenging moment. The more you use them, the stronger they will become. Each time you fall back on a principle, it's like sharpening your knives. Soon, you will have a set of razor-sharp tools always at the ready.

> You have the power to decide how you want to feel.

We are often so wrapped up in one way
of thinking that we don't have the
freedom to see ourselves any other way.
Developing the ability to use your own
insight to step outside of your experience
is the gift of perspective.

Chapter Four

THE FIRST PRINCIPLE
PERSPECTIVE

A RUSSIAN DANCE COACH ONCE SAID TO ME IN HIS BROKEN ENGLISH, "In order to be successful, you must see your dancing on the inside and outside at the same time." He told me that many dancers don't learn to dance as freely and as fully as they could until they retire. At that point, they're able to step outside of their own experience and take in their performances as the audience had been doing for decades. But by then, with an aged body, it's too late. Simply stated: Hindsight is 20/20. When the moment has passed, it's too late to relive it.

What he was really talking about is perspective. To me, this means being able to pendulate between the emotions and passions of being fully inside your life experiences while retaining the ability to step outside of yourself and see the whole reality clearly before things get overwhelming. When you look at things from the outside, it helps you to separate yourself from them momentarily and make better decisions. This is true for both the big things—your family, your job, your relationships, your dreams—as well as the smaller, more fleeting moments and interactions that make up your day-to-day life.

We are always given signs that something needs to change, that we need to see ourselves from the inside and outside at the same time. The bad news? We don't always appreciate those signs, and ignoring them can have devastating results. I had been ignoring my body's cries for help for years before my hip finally gave out. I had been working too much, not resting enough, and generally pushing myself above and beyond my physical capacity for decades. From my perch at the top of a lesson hard-earned, I can see that I blatantly ignored the messages my body was giving me for years. I so desperately wanted to believe that my body could handle anything I asked of it that I broke myself in the process. I was stuck in one way of perceiving things, in one belief of how things should be, which made me unable to step out of my own experience and see myself from the outside, to zoom out and see the bigger picture. If I had been able to gain perspective, I would have seen a young woman who was dangerously close to injuring herself permanently.

Breaking my hip and being forced to open my yoga studio in a wheelchair was the greatest teaching moment of my life, and the most humbling. I wouldn't trade it, but if I were given a do-over, an opportunity to take a time machine back to that period of my life, I would definitely loosen the steely grip I had on my hard-and-fast beliefs—that I should be at a certain level of fitness, that I should have a certain amount of stamina, that I should have a specific tolerance to pain. Now, at the first sign of discomfort, I try to really listen. I think of it like being tapped gently on the shoulder by someone who desperately needs your attention. At first the tapping is soft, maybe with one delicate finger: *Tap tap tap, please pay attention to this thing that needs to change.* But if you ignore the tap, it eventually turns into a push, which turns into a shove, and then, before you know it, you've been right-hooked by this thing that needs to change, by this new viewpoint that needs to be taken.

Thankfully, crisis isn't the only way to broaden your perspective. As human beings we are given countless chances to experiment with this fundamental principle. I see this in my own life every day. Whether it's in my relationship with my husband, when I'm parenting my kids, in the choices I make around food and exercise, in how I work or how I play, I always have the option to click into perspective, to use it as a path to living the life I want to live. From the moment I open my eyes in the morning until the moment I close them at night, I experience hundreds of opportunities to use this principle—and now I know better than to ignore them.

How many times have you looked back at a situation wishing you'd behaved differently? For a large part of my life, I was very reactive and had a lot of rage. I'd respond

Perspective through the Body

Of all the Living Clearly Principles, perspective is the one that lives primarily in the realm of the head. It requires a deliberate shifting of your mind-set, a rational decision to alter the way you're perceiving a situation to take in a wider view of it or to get into another person's experience. When you activate perspective, you start to think about things from another angle. Instead of hyperfocusing on one point (*Sleeping in will feel so good; it's warm and cozy in my bed, and going for a run will require that I leave it*), you activate the Perspective Process (page 36) to take in a broader view of the situation. The more you practice, the harder it will be to remain rigid in one way of seeing things. Your field of vision will naturally broaden, whether you like it or not (*But I feel so good after I run; I'm more awake and energized for the day; running helps me maintain a weight that feels right, that helps me feel good in my new jeans*).

Like everything about Living Clearly, perspective must be experienced through the body for it to become an established part of who you are. The Activation and Release exercise (page 40) and the Yoga for Perspective sequence (page 46) are excellent ways to physically experience how tension takes over the body and then dissolves, takes over and dissolves, just like any challenge you meet and then move through. And you can practice activating and releasing anywhere; you don't have to do the specific sequences listed in the book. Just clench your jaw, make tight fists, activate the muscles in your quads and glutes—and then release. You can do this while stuck in traffic, while waiting on line at the bank, when your computer is frozen, or even when you're on hold.

to people and situations angrily, and then feel guilty for weeks afterward. When I started practicing perspective, I gained more control over my reactions, which resulted in more pleasant interactions, fewer altercations, and significantly less guilt and regrets. Using perspective gives you instant hindsight.

One spring afternoon when I was pregnant with Rafael, Alec and I took Carmen out to the playground. I pushed the stroller with my big pregnant belly in tow. We talked and laughed as we walked down the street. As we approached a corner, a woman nearly

Chair Pose

When you're smack in the middle of a challenging moment—when the longing for chocolate has a death grip on you, when you're absolutely enraged by an e-mail you received at work, or when your 2-year-old has flung her body across a busy stretch of sidewalk because she wants a snack right now now now!—time seems to stand still. It can feel claustrophobic and deeply stressful, pushing you to wonder if you have what it takes to get through it. You do. You are stronger and more capable than you realize, and as you practice perspective (see the Perspective Process, page 36), you will be increasingly able to zoom out and see that this challenging moment is just one of zillions of moments that you'll experience in your lifetime: hard ones, happy ones, peaceful ones, agitating ones. Moments come and they go. Yoga poses can help you keep this in mind, especially challenging ones like Chair Pose. You can practice Chair Pose any time during the day—no yoga mat required. It's a wonderful way to light up the legs and fire up the core, more energizing than a late-afternoon cup of coffee, even. When you commit to the pose, exerting the muscular effort to firmly "sit" on that invisible chair, you are asking your quads and glutes—and shoulders and core, for that matter—to show up and strut their stuff. It can be hard. As you sit down as low as you can go and reach your arms out and up from your shoulders, hands reaching toward the sky, you may find yourself shaking, ticking off the seconds until the torture is over, but when it's over, and it will be over (everything is temporary), you will be filled with physical relief, yes, but also a clear sense of accomplishment and appreciation for all that your body can do—all that you can do.

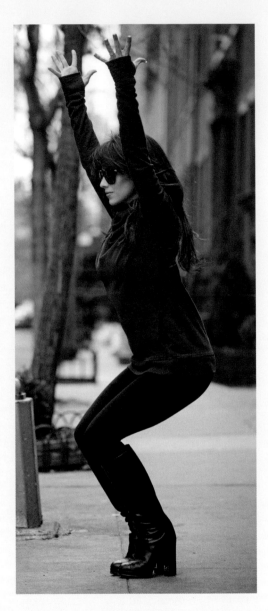

collided with Carmen's stroller. She looked at me, rolled her eyes, and said some not-so-yogic words loud enough for Carmen to hear. I was surprised, but in an effort to diffuse the situation, I simply said, "Thank you."

Well, that made her furious, and she launched into an angry rant about how I nearly crushed her foot with Carmen's stroller. I'll admit that it was pretty tanklike—many strollers are these days—but we were walking slowly and carefully. I smiled sweetly at her, pointed to my daughter, and indicated that this wasn't an appropriate way to speak in front of little Carmen. Well, that enraged her even more, and she responded with, "I get that you have a baby, and I get that you're pregnant, but you can't just push your stroller anywhere you want!" At this point, I realized that she wasn't going to calm down, so we turned and walked away.

My mama-bear instinct was to take the stroller, without my daughter in it, of course, and whack her with it. My perspective-powered approach, however, gave me the space to realize that this situation probably had very little do with us and everything to do with this woman's personal demons. I thought of the quote: "Be kind, for everyone you meet is fighting a battle you know nothing about." In that moment of space created through perspective, I was able to remind myself that I had no idea what this woman was dealing with in her own life. She could be having the worst day of her life. Tempered with this broader view of the situation, I understood that the worst thing I could do for myself and my family was feed off her stress and take it on as my own.

"Be kind, for everyone you meet is fighting a battle you know nothing about."

When you're in conflict with someone, you may not realize that you're in a deeply reactive space until you get to the part where you have to say you're sorry. In the moment, you're so heated up, your ego is raging, your blood is boiling, and you just can't stop your reactivity. It's like a boulder rolling down a hill: It starts slow, but as it builds momentum, it can't be stopped. You feel hurt, insulted, or wronged, and before you know it, you're yelling, saying hurtful things and slamming doors. Finding perspective means allowing ourselves to acknowledge that our feelings or attitudes toward a certain situation—or certain person—may shift once the drama has passed and our nervous system has calmed and our triggers are no longer activated.

THE PERSPECTIVE PROCESS

Perspective gives us a chance to ask, *How do I want this to go?* And in the space we create by asking that question, we can influence the course of events. But what is perspective, exactly? It's commonly defined as a specific point of view or a way of seeing something. There can be multiple perspectives on a given situation (if you need examples of that, check out our politicians). But for me, it's—unsurprisingly!—more active than that. Sure, perspective is something that happens, but only if *you* decide you want it to. There's innately some momentum behind it, some *umph* and focused attention; it's not a passive state of being.

The first step to bringing more perspective into your life is acknowledging that you need it. If you sense that you're more reactive than responsive (like if you find yourself spending more time apologizing for things you've said or done than you'd like to), or if you're dominated by feelings of worry or anxiety, or if you feel generally stuck and stagnant in your body, job, relationship, home life, anything, you could probably use some more perspective. And I've got a simple four-step process to get you there. To practice perspective and start the process of defusing reactivity and increasing your ability to hear what's really going on with yourself and others: 1) Pause. 2) Zoom out. 3) Reframe the situation with a key question. 4) Choose a new direction.

The next time you feel the stress rising—if your body is aching, if your heart is hurting, if your child is testing your patience or your partner is testing your compassion—bust out the perspective 1-2-3-4.

❶ Pause

It starts with a pause. This is the muscular aspect of the Perspective Process. In the beginning, it takes strength to slow the reactivity train. When your emotions have been in the driver's seat for a lifetime, they can easily snowball, quickly gaining speed and momentum. Most of us are like puppets being manipulated by our strong and reactive feelings. At the first inkling of hurt, craving, anger, frustration, disappointment, or sadness, we give up and allow ourselves to be tossed around by our emotions. But when we pause just for a moment—it can be as brief as 2 seconds—we create a subtle but powerful space that allows for a fork in the road where there was once only one direction to go. The next time you feel your defenses rise or notice that you are longing for

Savasana for Perspective

Sometimes perspective is about zooming in. There are moments in our lives when it's necessary to temper the distractions that pull us out of ourselves, the ones that make our minds fuzzy and our hearts anxious. When the busy monkey mind begins to stand still, we have access to great reserves of peace and well-being and are able to hear the often quiet but essential directives of the body. Savasana, or Corpse Pose, is a wonderful way to practice leaving the outside world behind. Life doesn't stop when you decide to get quiet. Can you stay focused in the midst of the storm? Savasana traditionally comes at the end of a yoga class, but as an exercise to practice perspective, I recommend taking a short Corpse Pose any time you need a reboot in the middle of the day—it can be 2 minutes or 20, or longer if you have time. All you need is a clean place to get flat on your back. This could be on your child's floor while she's napping, on your office floor (it helps to close your door), or in your living room or bedroom.

The first step in assuming Savasana is to lie flat on the floor or other supportive surface. Once you're there, focus on releasing your body into the ground. Here, gravity is working for you. Allow the floor to hold you firmly; sink into it fully. Scan your body from the tips of your fingers to the ends of your toes. Whenever you come upon a place of tension, exhale and let it go. Allow yourself to take in the sounds around you. You may hear sirens, cars driving by, dogs barking. Take in the noises you hear, and then begin to drop them one by one by creating a separation between you and the sounds—you are not the sounds and the sounds are not you. You are here, in this body, on this mat, on the floor (you may be on your office carpet, and that's perfectly okay). Keep coming back to the sensations in your body. Feel your torso, arms, and legs sinking into the ground; feel the back of your head cradled by this firm foundation. If your mind has left the room, following the auditory bread crumbs of a noisy garbage truck or a crying baby, call it back to the refuge of your body, creating space between you and the outside world.

something or someone, practice catching yourself in the moment before you take action. By simply recognizing that you are experiencing strong feelings, you reclaim the pause and regain the ability to alter the course of events. To be clear, I'm not suggesting that you stop feeling what you're feeling. You're not trying to stuff a cork back into an already popped bottle of champagne. You want to maintain your passion, but just like a bottle of bubbly that's opened slowly and thoughtfully, you can acknowledge the emotions you're experiencing without them exploding all over the place. That acknowledgment is the pause.

② Zoom Out

Once you've steadied yourself with the pause, you're ready for the next step in the Perspective Process, zooming out. Just like a camera, we have the ability to hone in on the tiniest details of a situation—often our own feelings about what's happening—or to zoom out and take in more of what's actually transpiring, which includes the other person's experience and what things could possibly look like once the moment is over. Zooming out is the heart of perspective. When we pause and then zoom out, it's like we are hovering above the situation, empowered with the gift of broad-reaching sight.

This part of the Perspective Process makes me think of Maria, a student who came to me for private sessions. She was 34 and pregnant with her first child. Though she was filled with happy anticipation about meeting her baby, she also seemed angry, agitated, and just generally "off." After working closely together for some time, she eventually opened up to me about what was troubling her: road rage. Throughout her pregnancy— she was 4 months along when we started working together—she often found herself boiling with anger when she was behind the wheel. When people would tailgate or cut her off—par for the course in New York City—she reacted furiously. If someone was following her too closely, she would slow down dramatically, forcing them to slow down, too. She would also give them the finger or wave condescendingly. Maria attributed a lot of it to the ping-ponging hormones of pregnancy, but she no longer wanted to be a slave to her reactivity. She hoped that there was something we could do together that would help her find more peace when she was driving.

My first job was to help Maria and her baby stay safe. I did this by encouraging her to zoom out and remember that cars aren't made of glass, therefore you cannot see within, and that they are driven by an actual person with a life and a family. I asked her if she could use perspective to begin to shift the way she was envisioning the driver. Could she, from her newly zoomed out position, treat the other person the way she wanted to be treated? I reminded Maria that her own anger increased her chances of getting into an accident—strong emotions are distracting and discombobulating. Zooming out would also help her see that succumbing to rage could have devastating effects on her life and the life of her unborn child.

❸ Reframe the Situation with a Key Question

Once you've paused and zoomed out, it's time to reframe the situation with a key question. In Maria's case, I asked her to consider the possible consequences of following through with her anger. I had her ask, *What could happen to me, or my baby, if I followed through with my rage?* Together, we explored possible consequences. If Maria slammed on her brakes when someone was tailgating her, the other driver could rear-end her vehicle aggressively, setting off her airbags, giving her whiplash, or worse. If she made an antagonistic gesture to a driver who was enraging her, like giving the finger or waving condescendingly, she could end up in a heated altercation, which could raise her blood pressure and leave her shaken—not good for a growing baby. These possible outcomes gave Maria serious pause. She was beginning to see just how harmful her road rage could be.

Regardless of the challenge you're facing, it is always possible to ask a key question:

(continued on page 42)

Activation and Release

It's one thing to experience perspective, and it's another thing to feel it. When working one-on-one with clients, I help them become intimate with the sensations that come up in the body when faced with conflict of any kind. When you are challenged by anything—a rude comment, an aggressive driver, a desire for something you should probably resist (think: cheese fries, a cigarette, sleeping in instead of working out)—your body tenses up. Some common areas of tension are the jaw, neck, throat, face, shoulders, arms, hands, back, and legs. When you become familiar with the unique way your body reacts to stressors, you will be able to notice, more quickly and efficiently, when you are being challenged, which helps you avoid getting swept away in the emotion of the moment. I have my clients practice activation and release exercises to experience tension in a muscle or group of muscles and then see what it feels like when those muscles relax. A tensed muscle is a tensed muscle whether you are consciously exercising it or it is stressed. This is why it is extremely beneficial to learn how to activate and release your muscles in the safety of a controlled yoga environment—instead of on the highway or when your boss is yelling at you. If you can release a tensed muscle on your yoga mat, then you can learn to do the same thing in a tension-filled situation.

A 60-SECOND EXERCISE:
BICYCLE CRUNCHES TO CLAMSHELL CRUNCHES

To experience activation and release, you must work extremely hard for a burst (1 minute for this exercise) and then relax. For these 60 seconds, give it your all, push yourself as hard as you can. Then completely let go and notice how the burning sensation releases and your breath calms and resumes a regular pattern. You can do challenging things. Your body was designed to work like this. What felt impossible or insurmountable (60 seconds of full effort can feel like 1,000 seconds) is absolutely achievable, and when you face a challenge the next time, you'll remember that it won't last forever. Intense activation or effort followed by release is a beautiful representation of your ability to move through difficult circumstances that you encounter in life.

Set a timer for 1 minute. Do 10 Bicycle Crunches followed immediately by 10 Clamshell Crunches (for instructions, see pages 48 to 49 of the Yoga for Perspective sequence), and repeat the cycle for the full 60 seconds. As you get stronger, you'll be able to increase the time to 2 and then 3 minutes of consecutive Bicycle and Clamshell Crunches. When the timer goes off, stop. Lie flat on the floor. Inhale deeply until your body can't expand any more. Hold your breath, and then exhale with a big sigh through your mouth. Repeat the breathing cycle two more times. Place one hand on your belly and one hand on your chest. Notice how the burning in your abdomen starts to release and your breath regulates. After all of that effort, you sink into complete relief.

Bicycle Crunches

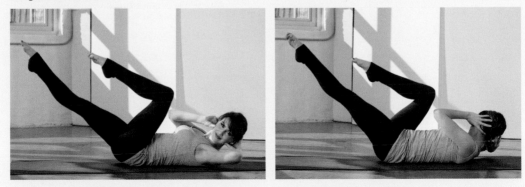

Clamshell Crunches

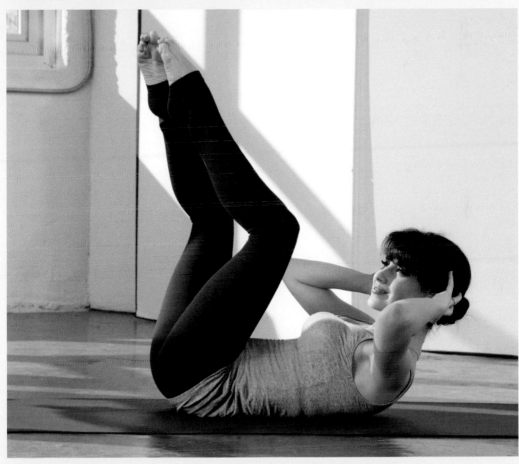

If I follow through with this current desire, how will I feel later or how will my life be influenced? A key question can also help you take in the scope of your life instead of honing in on one aspect that you're not that into—like your dress size, your relationship status, or the number in your checking account. You may also find that from your zoomed-out position, you can ask a question about the other person's experience, like, *What could it possibly feel like to be in her shoes?*

❹ Choose a New Direction

The fourth and final step of the Perspective Process is choosing a new direction. This is the fun part! This is where you really feel what it's like to steer your ship toward a bright and welcoming new land. *You* get to decide how you will navigate your way through a challenging moment, and how you'll feel after it's over. You are no longer dragged around by your emotions.

In my life, and I hear the same thing from moms all over the country, I find that my toddler is particularly adept at providing me with opportunities to practice Step 4 of the process. Even during the writing of this book, actually, *especially* during the writing of this book, little Carmen had me on my toes. Like most 2-year-olds, my daughter is the princess. She can be sweet and kind, but only when it is convenient to her. She's all

SAMPLE REFRAMING QUESTIONS

Reframing questions can look a lot of ways. Here are a few examples.

- ► How will I feel later this afternoon if I have a doughnut for breakfast?

- ► What will my stress levels be like tomorrow if I put off the work that I have to do today?

- ► What am I appreciative of right now, in this very moment?

- ► How will I feel later if I react angrily to my toddler's meltdown?

- ► What will screaming at my husband really accomplish?

- ► What could be happening in my friend's/sister's/mother's/child's life that is motivating her to act this way?

- ► How will my body feel if I skip my workout today?

smiles one minute and deep in a tantrum the next. And just like so many mothers I know, I juggle a lot. I'm a teacher, a mother to small children, a wife with a busy husband who wants me to participate in his life. In an ideal world, Carmen would understand this and cooperate when I need it most. But she's 2. And often does only what she wants, like 2-year-olds are developmentally designed to do. During a particularly busy stretch of writing and recipe testing, Carmen woke up from her nap to find her babysitter and my recipe developer, Melissa, in the kitchen with me. Whenever she has to share me with others, she gets territorial, and the message is clear: Don't take me away from my mommy. She just wanted me to hold her, and she cried and screamed if I spoke to anyone else or sat down or asked her if she wanted something to eat. She would yell, "*Mami, solo quiero abrazarte!*" Which is the sweetest thing: "Mommy, I only want to hug you." But she was trying to hit Melissa and her babysitter, and if they attempted to engage with her, she told them they were not allowed to talk to her. I know by now that the only way to diffuse a situation like this is to practice perspective. Instead of reacting negatively, I create the space to understand what is really going on in my child's experience.

> I know by now that the only way to diffuse a situation is to practice perspective.

So, I did. I paused in the middle of her tantrum, zoomed out to see what was really happening, and asked two key questions: *How will I feel if I lose my temper and yell at my daughter* (guilty, sad, remorseful) and *What does it feel like to be Carmen right now?* In doing so, I realized that this is a big moment for her. She is only 2 years old, and even an hour or two away from her mother can seem like an eternity. While I could see that the situation really was no big deal, that her outing with her babysitter and her nap only took her away from me for a few hours and that our guests would be leaving soon, giving us some cozy alone time before dinner, she can't yet grasp concepts like time, so this intrusion into her home space felt like a very big deal. While I wished that she would quietly eat a snack and play with her toys so I could talk to the adults, I imagined what it was like to be in her little shoes and understood that teaching her about healthy separation is a slow and gentle process. With this perspective, I was able to see that she very soon won't want to be with me constantly like she does now. Before I know it, she'll be slamming doors and telling me to go away. I know that I want to hold on to these sweet moments as long as possible. And while I needed to work, I saw that the only way

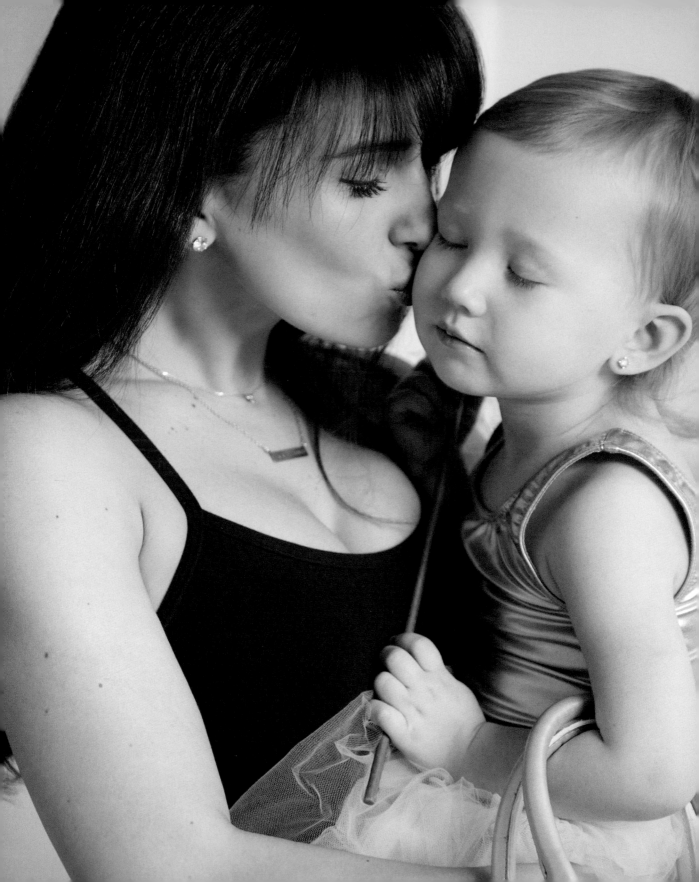

to get there was to meet her on her level. So instead of reacting, I chose a new direction. I hugged her, and I breathed myself into releasing any frustration that I was feeling. Taking the time to be calm on the front end would give me more time to work later. I kept my body relaxed and my voice soft. I colored and played with her toys until my calmness took over and she joined me. Soon she was playing on her own, and I was able to get to work.

By understanding that we each have our own point of view—even 2-year-olds see things in their own unique way—we open ourselves up to deeper connections with others, increasing our empathy and compassion and bridging the gap that feeds misunderstanding and misalignment. By pulling the camera back and disentangling ourselves from a micro view of a situation, we liberate ourselves from the confines of a singular point of view. Things no longer have to look one way to be good or right. Perspective helps us understand that we respond differently when we are caught in the hurricane of emotionality.

Now, steadied with perspective, you are ready to move into the next principle, to slow down and fill your body with the transformative power of breathing. Let's go!

The Wisdom of Heartbreak

Sometimes perspective is a journey that has a beginning, middle, and end. For this, I always think of heartbreak. Heartbreak is a fundamental component of human development, but when we are in its grasp, it is incredibly painful. We can't sleep, eat, or smile, and the whole world seems gloomy and pointless. But then time passes and we move on. We look back from our newly healed perspective almost surprised at how much we were once hurting. Healed and rejuvenated, proudly bearing scar tissue in our hearts, it's easy to wonder if all that heartache was really worth it. The next time you're in the throes of emotional upheaval, when your heart hurts so much it truly feels like it will shatter into a million tiny pieces, hang tight, keep moving forward day by day, taking baby steps toward a brighter destination. Perspective is being able to understand that this too shall pass.

YOGA FOR PERSPECTIVE

There are opportunities to practice perspective at every moment of a yoga class, but it is in the challenging moments, like holding a dynamic Chair Pose or doing Bicycle Crunches, that we benefit from pulling back and taking in the broader scope of our experiences. Chair Pose is challenging, but your body is designed to carry you through this pose with more ease than you can imagine. You think you can't do it, but there you are, doing it! Give yourself more credit, and enjoy what your body is capable of achieving. *Approximately 15 minutes*

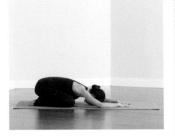

1 Start in **CHILD'S POSE**. Move your hips back to the heels, and bring your forehead to the mat with your arms framing your head, palms facing down. Let your elbows sink into the floor, allowing the shoulder blades to release away from your thoracic spine, the weight of each blade melting down into your upper arms and into the elbows. Allow your forehead to move gently from side to side while the sit bones release down toward your heels. There should be no tension in your shoulders, brow, jaw, or face. Your body should be perfectly at ease, in a completely inactive state except for the ebbing and flowing of your breath.

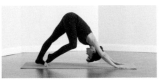

2 Softness turns into action as you extend through your fingertips and rise up into **DOWNWARD FACING DOG**. Gently peddle your feet out and allow your hips to go from side to side. Throughout, notice the shift of perspective from soft to active.

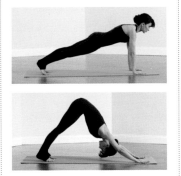

3 Inhale forward into **PLANK POSE**, shoulders over your wrists, heels reaching backward. Exhale back into **DOWNWARD FACING DOG**.

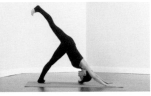
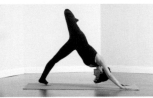
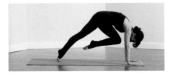

4 Inhale your right leg up into **DOWNWARD FACING DOG SPLIT**. Exhale open your hip, turning your leg out and bending your right knee. Inhale straighten, extend, and reach your leg back into Downward Facing Dog Split, squaring your hips to the floor. Exhale, activate your core, round your spine, and bring your shoulders over your wrists as you bring your right knee to your nose. Inhale long and strong back into Downward Facing Dog Split. Exhale, activate your center, and guide your right knee to your right triceps, with your shoulders perfectly aligned over your wrists. Inhale back into Downward Facing Dog Split. Exhale twist through your center as you bring your right knee across to touch your left triceps, your shoulders moving past your wrists. Inhale return to a squared off (hips parallel with the floor) Downward Facing Dog Split.

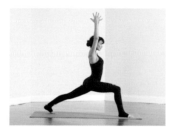

5 Exhale your right foot all the way between your hands. Inhale raise your torso up into a **HIGH LUNGE**. Exhale, soften, and settle into the pose, shoulders down your back, knee over your ankle.

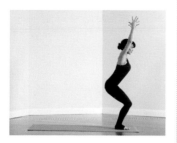

6 Inhale step your left foot forward to meet your right, your toes and heels touching, coming into **CHAIR POSE**. Exhale, bring your feet together, and sit down deeply, relaxing your shoulders, extending long and strong through your elbows. With every single inhale find strength, and with every single exhale find softness. This pose is the perfect example of practicing activation and release in one asana, asking us to embrace perspective in every moment of the pose. Take five rounds of breath here.

7 Inhale, step your left foot back into **HIGH LUNGE**, straighten your spine, and soften your shoulders.

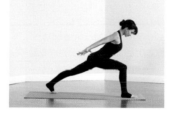

8 Exhale, tip your body weight forward at a 45-degree angle, and reach your arms straight out behind you into little airplane wings, palms facing downward, with a strong, straight back leg. Feel your front leg firing up. As you note how challenging this posture feels, use the **PERSPECTIVE PROCESS** to remind yourself that everything is temporary. Take five rounds of breath here.

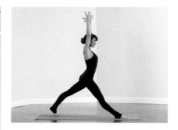

9 Inhale stretch your arms over your head as you lift your torso back into **HIGH LUNGE** and straighten your front knee for a little relief from the burn you have collected in your quads. Exhale rebend your right knee back over your ankle.

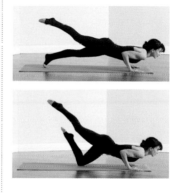

10 Inhale, place your hands on either side of your foot, and move into **PLANK POSE** with an option to lift your right leg (you can also drop your left knee to the floor to create more ease). Feel how your core fires up. You are shifting the work from one part of your body to another, creating a balanced workout.

(continued)

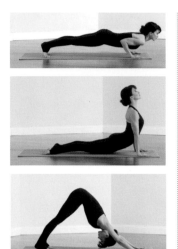

⓫ Exhale into **CHATURANGA**, inhale **UPWARD FACING DOG**, and exhale **DOWNWARD FACING DOG**.

⓬ Inhale your left leg up into **DOWNWARD FACING DOG SPLIT**. Exhale open up your hip. Inhale your leg long and strong behind you. Exhale your knee to your nose, shoulders over your wrists, and inhale your leg long. Exhale your knee to your left triceps, activating your core, and inhale your leg long **DOWNWARD FACING DOG SPLIT**. Exhale your knee across your body to your right triceps and inhale your leg back long behind you.

⓭ Exhale step your foot between your hands. Inhale up into **HIGH LUNGE**, bringing your arms up and softening the shoulders down your back. Exhale, strengthen your back leg, and focus on

your front leg as it starts to heat up.

⓮ Inhale, using your core to draw your right leg in to meet your left in **CHAIR POSE**. Exhale soften into the posture, finding strength and softness. Take five rounds of breath.

⓯ Inhale step your right foot back into **HIGH LUNGE**, straightening your torso up and softening your shoulders down your back.

⓰ Exhale, tip your body weight forward, and bring your airplane arms straight out behind you, palms down, with a strong, straight back leg. Feel the heat and the challenge and use perspective to sense how this feeling is temporary, how it is building strength in your body. Take five rounds of breath here.

⓱ Inhale return to **HIGH LUNGE**, reaching your arms up and straightening your front leg. Exhale rebend your front knee.

⓲ Inhale, place your hands on either side of your foot, moving into **PLANK POSE** with an option to lift your left leg (you can place your right knee on the floor to create more ease).

⓳ Exhale **CHATURANGA**, inhale **UPWARD FACING DOG**, and exhale **DOWNWARD FACING DOG**.

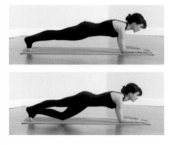

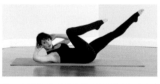

⓴ Inhale into **PLANK POSE**, but this time bring your feet together. Exhale lower down onto your forearms, coming into **DOLPHIN PLANK**. Make sure your pelvis is parallel with the floor, firing up your core. This is a difficult pose (fantastic for toning your abs) always remember that the fiery sensation is temporary and you can totally do it. Jog the knees for 10 counts, breathing in and out steadily.

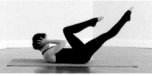

㉑ Inhale straighten both legs back into a strong **DOLPHIN PLANK** for one breath, exhale, release down to your mat, and flip over onto your back for core work. Bring your knees up and begin opposite elbow, opposite knee **BICYCLE CRUNCHES** for 20 counts.

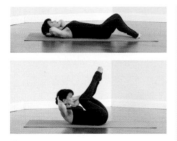

22 Transition to **CLAM CRUNCHES**, knees butterflied open, soles of your feet touching, and hands interlaced behind your head. Inhale to prepare, and then exhale, lift the torso, bringing your elbows toward your knees while trying to touch them together. Inhale back down. Repeat 10 times.

23 Do **BICYCLE CRUNCHES** for 10 counts.

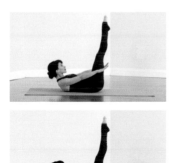

24 Move into **100 VARIATIONS**, legs straight up, arms long next to your body. Inhale to prepare, exhale lift your shoulders, neck, and head toward your legs, pulsing up for 10 counts. Then micro pulse your arms quickly up and down for 10 counts.

25 Do **BICYCLE CRUNCHES** for 10 counts.

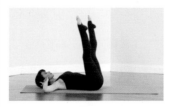

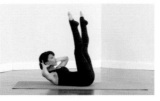

26 Transition into **STRADDLE UPS**, legs straight up, feet 2 feet apart. Inhale to prepare, exhale lift your chest and pelvis off your mat toward one another, using your core muscles and rounding the spine. Inhale, release down, exhale, repeat. Do 10 reps.

27 Do **BICYCLE CRUNCHES** for 10 counts.

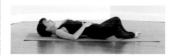

28 Rest on your back with one hand on your belly and one on your chest. Remind yourself that it is over and that you are okay. It is easy to move into a state of fight-or-flight when we are worked up. Bring yourself back into a state of centeredness and calm by reminding yourself that you are no longer doing the exercise. Notice your

heartbeat, notice your pulse. See that they are beating at the same pace, which is probably very fast. Take a deep breath, expanding your belly as big as possible into a Buddha belly, hold the breath at its peak, sip in another bit of air, and then exhale audibly and fully. We can go from a very active state to a total released state, which is our practice of perspective; we are living one way and then can transition to a completely different way. As you inhale, scan your body for any tension. When you exhale, let go of that tension, reminding yourself that all those burning sensations were temporary.

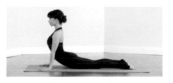

29 Take a deep inhale, flip onto your tummy, and exhale. Place your hands on your mat toward the bottom of your rib cage and inhale into **HIGH COBRA**.

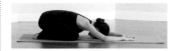

30 Exhale return to **CHILD'S POSE**. Notice how different you feel in this pose after your practice. See where you worked your body. Feel the tingle in your thighs and your core. Sense the pace of your breath and the sweat on your skin.

From the first faint breath of the infant to the last gasp of the dying man . . . life is but a series of breaths.

—YOGI RAMACHARAKA, *SCIENCE OF BREATH*

Chapter Five

THE SECOND PRINCIPLE
BREATHING

YOU'RE RUNNING LATE FOR WORK. YOU HAD A HUGE FIGHT WITH YOUR partner over who forgot to take out the garbage. Perhaps your 3-year-old threw himself on the floor every time you said "shoes," and you had to carry him barefoot and screaming to the car. Whatever the reason, there's no way you're going to make it on time today. This reality has your mind blitzing with uncomfortable scenarios: You're imagining your coworkers sneering as you tiptoe to your desk or the talking-to your boss will deliver later in the day. There will be no time for coffee or breakfast, and you wonder if you can run in heels. Your head is pounding with what-ifs and oh-nos, and your body is responding in turn. Your shoulders are hunched, brow furrowed, jaw clenched. You feel sweat pooling in your underarms, your heart is slamming in your chest, and your breath is short and tight in your throat. You feel out of control, anxious, and panicked— hopeless, really.

Then, miraculously, you summon the inner strength to pause and take a deep breath. This momentary lull in the action, this tiny interruption—it can be 10 seconds or even just 2—activates the Perspective Process. Before you know it, you're seeing the big(ger) picture. Your new vantage point allows you to take in the entirety of what's going on here: You have allowed your mind to hijack your experience, and your body is being dragged along for the panicky ride. From up here, at the 10,000-foot view of perspective, you remember that you're a strong member of your team at work, that you're efficient and productive, and that even if you are tardy occasionally, your work doesn't suffer. You'll make up for it by eating lunch at your desk or staying late from time to time. The boiling pot of your stress response is beginning to simmer. Deep breath.

Now your line of vision is getting even wider. You can see that all this nervous energy is just feeding more nervous energy and that stress begets stress. You understand that allowing worry to overcome you narrowed your focus so significantly that your experience was made up of nothing but the hypothetical disasters your mind was conjuring up. And that's a dangerously myopic place to be. Your body was contracted and rigid, your breath short and shallow; you were a petri dish for tension. You realize that all this stress and fretting does nothing to help you get to work on time.

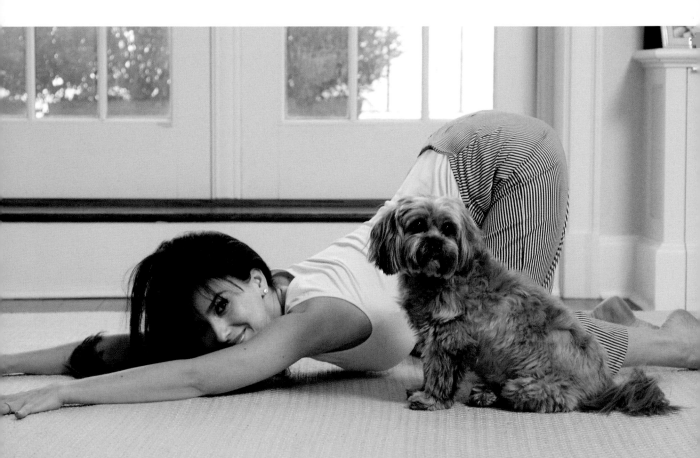

With perspective on your side, you're ready to sweeten your experience by turning to the second principle, breathing. With just a bit of attention and intention—and the willingness to practice—you will find breath can quickly become your steady companion as you travel along the path to Living Clearly. I love teaching students about mindful breathing because it is a resource that every human being has access to. The breath is there for us in every moment, anywhere: at the post office, with your children, during a meeting, while driving. You don't need to learn a complex fitness routine, buy fancy workout clothes, find your sneakers, or carve out 90 minutes. Whether you are older or younger, are in shape or out of shape, have tons of free time or barely any downtime, the breath is always there—and it's yours for the taking.

Breath is the bridge that connects life to consciousness, the bridge that unites your body to your thoughts. Whenever your mind becomes scattered, use your breath as the means to take hold of your mind again.

—THICH NHAT HANH

Your lungs work hard all day to bring fresh supplies of oxygen to your body and to rid it of carbon dioxide, a waste product. About 12 to 20 times per minute, your lungs—teaming up with the muscular output of your diaphragm—expand and contract in the elegant dance that is breathing. This effort goes relatively unnoticed by most of us, but once you begin to bring your awareness to what your breath is doing in any given moment, you will start to see patterns, to draw connections between the emotions you are experiencing and how you are breathing. This is the first step toward mindful breathing, or getting the breath to work for you. At any given moment, you can check in with your breath, and it will have a good amount of information for you.

Try it now. Put this book down and bring awareness to how you are breathing. Is your breath short and quick? Or is it deep and steady? Are your breaths shallow, only filling a bit of your lungs? Or are you breathing to full capacity? And what about your belly? Is it expanding with the inhale and contracting with exhale? Note how you're breathing, and then, for fun, try something different. If your breath is choppy, focus on completing a smooth inhale and exhale. Steady the breath. Imagine that it's a gentle breeze flowing into you and out of you—soft, easy, no rough edges or snags. Practice this easy, steady breath for 1 minute, and see how it makes you feel. You'll probably find that your heart rate slows and your mind starts to relax. Now play with the opposite. Hold your breath for a few counts, and then take short, sharp, fast breaths. Notice the way your body contracts and how your mind gets busy.

All stress starts and ends with the breath. When we are under pressure of any kind, we stop breathing—note what happens to your breath when you're rushed, scared, surprised, or angry (it stops). And when the breath returns, it's usually choppy, uncoordinated, shallow, and incomplete. This kind of unfocused breathing reminds me of the work I did with Brian, a client who came to me hoping to deepen his yoga practice. Brian was good-looking and charming with a high-powered job. He'd always show up 15 minutes late to my group classes and flash a beaming smile that would make anyone forgive him for asking them to move their mats around midclass. He would often stay after my class to ask questions about what I taught that day or to get a few minutes of focused attention on his handstands—an overachieving type, for sure.

All stress starts and ends with the breath.

I eventually agreed to work with him privately and quickly learned that the work he needed to do had nothing to do with inversions. Our one-on-one sessions would take place at his apartment in Manhattan, and he was always running late— texting me, making excuses, asking me to wait just 10 more minutes. At the beginning of our work together, I would tack on extra time at the end of each session to give him a full hour. But after a month of steady lateness, I changed my tune, stopping our sessions when they were scheduled to end. He was surprised but gracious, and I told him that if we started on time, he could, of course, have the full hour. During the course of 5 months working together, I learned that his ongoing tardiness to my group classes and his incessant lateness for our private sessions were not unique to his work with me. I discovered that being late was the thread that ran through every part of his life: He was always a few steps behind, missing important deadlines and appointments. His charm and easygoing manner helped him dodge accountability. He was good at what he did, so his company did not want to lose him. He was a sweet person, so his friends would wait around for him to show up to dinner or parties. But even if he wasn't directly experiencing the consequences of his tardiness, his chronic lateness was taking a toll on his work, relationships, and stress levels. He was in a continuous state of anxiety—heart racing, breath constricted, shoulders hunched.

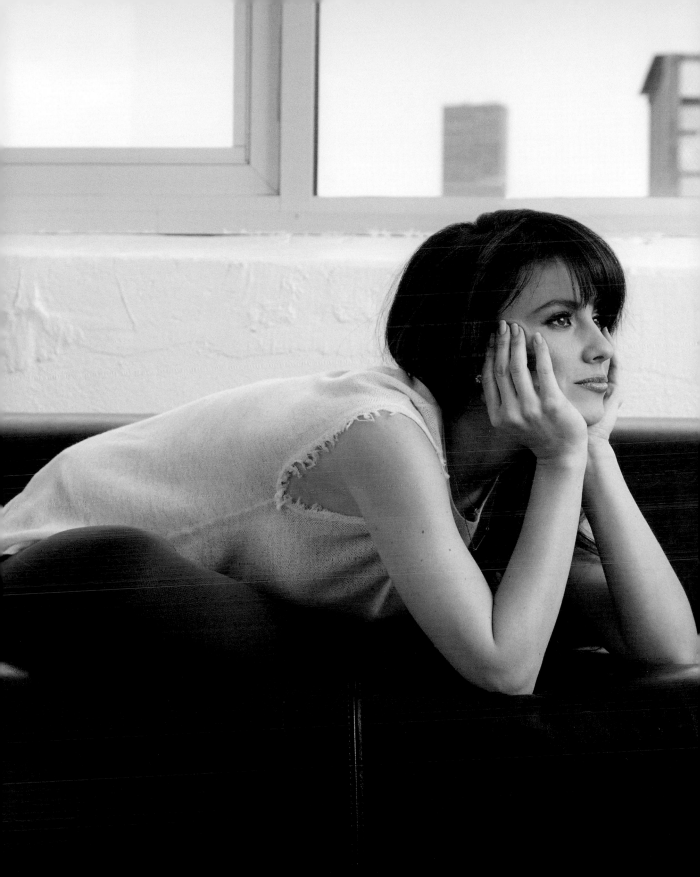

A Simple Breath: Sama Vritti

Sama Vritti, or equal breathing, is one of the easiest breathing practices. In Sanskrit, *sama* means "even, smooth, or flat" and *vritti* means "fluctuations or modifications," and together the phrase refers to the technique of calming the mental fluctuations of the mind—the anxiety, worries, fears, insecurities, and regrets that we all carry—through a smooth and even breath. I always recommend that beginner students start out with this breath because it is easy to practice (you can do it anywhere without drawing attention to yourself) but also has a deceptively challenging aspect that must be addressed to fully experience the benefits of mindful breathing. I use this breath when I feel anger begin to flare up or when I'm asked to navigate a challenging situation, like facing a crowd of paparazzi outside my apartment building while trying to get two kids out the door in the morning.

As you begin to practice this breath, you may notice that it is significantly easier to inhale than it is to exhale. This is because we are programmed to avoid suffocation at all costs, and so we are hyperfocused on bringing air into the body. As you experiment with Sama Vritti, pay close attention to the out-breath, aiming for longer, slower exhalations. The length of the inhale must be the same as the length of the exhale. Focus on emptying your lungs completely, as if you are squeezing all the air out of a balloon. If you bring your attention to the exhale, the inhale will take care of itself. This practice is the pathway to steady, regulated, complete breathing. Think of weight training. When you do a complete biceps curl, you bring the weight all the way to your shoulder and all the way down until your arm is fully extended. A full range of motion has a beginning, middle, and end. It's the same with the breath. A full range of motion with the breath is not complete until you have exhaled completely.

See page 68 of the Yoga for Breathing sequence for detailed instructions on practicing Sama Vritti. Keeping track of your breathing counts can be helpful with this exercise. You can download a metronome app on your phone, or you can tap out the counts on a table or your thigh.

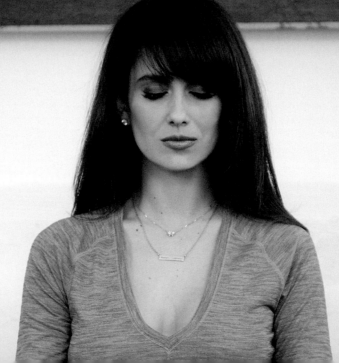

And one day, his composure collapsed; he was no longer able to keep all that anxiety at bay. That morning, he raced to JFK to make a flight to Dallas for an important meeting. He made it just in time, lucky as always, only to discover that his flight was taking off from LaGuardia Airport, 40 minutes away. Ah! He called me from the airport in a full state of panic, asking if I had time for a session later that day. I did, and when I arrived at his apartment, he was on his front stoop in tears. He jumped up when he saw me and gave me a huge, sobbing hug. Here was this handsome, successful man, clinging to this small yoga instructor on Eighth Street. I walked him into his apartment and sat him down. His place was a disaster: I stepped over piles of papers, CDs, and clothes and got him a glass of water from the kitchen. Then we began the practice.

When I moved him into Savasana, the opening pose, he was still sobbing. I guided him through noticing his breath, grounding, finding his center, and finally letting go. At this point, he was able to tell me what happened at the airport. Turns out he didn't lose his job that day, but he did lose his cool. This had happened before, he said, when he missed important meetings, but this was the first time he was honest with himself about the debilitating panic that set in when he was late—which was most of the time.

From that day forward, we worked closely with his breath. I helped him see that he held his breath whenever he was running late and when he started to breathe again, it would be choppy and shallow. The lateness plus the disrupted breathing fed upon each other until he disconnected from himself completely. He was so emotionally charged and physically tense that he ended up in a full-blown panic attack.

We practiced simple breathing exercises like Sama Vritti (opposite) that he could do anywhere to calm his racing mind and relax his heart. I couldn't directly influence his lateness, but I could give him tools that would help him decrease stress in those high-intensity moments. And through our work together, he eventually faced the fact that he was overtaxed by his high-pressure job, an uncomfortable truth that caused him to emotionally "check out" from what was happening in the present moment. This checked-out or foggy state led to his chronic tardiness. By creating healthier boundaries at work, he slowly started to feel more whole and less depleted, which, of course, helped him become more punctual.

THE UNEXPECTED POWER OF THE BREATH

When we hold the breath, we move quickly into fight-or-flight mode: We contract, react, or flee. With the breath constricted, we are resistant and not in touch with our higher self, the place from which we can make wise decisions. But when we create the space for even a few mindful breaths in a stressful situation, we have access to the softer and more intuitive aspects of ourselves and become more compassionate, forgiving, and empathic. With breath on your side, you become alert and aware of what's really going on, not overtaken by ego, old stories, and destructive patterns. You can see clearly.

When we breathe mindfully, we initiate a response in the body that moves us out of the stress state and into a more relaxed place. The first step in the shift is recategorizing breath. While breathing is indeed an obvious function of our physical makeup, the way we breathe can also be consciously controlled to bring about a desired change in our mental and physical states. And while breathing is a vehicle for the oxygen that nourishes our cells, the breath that moves in and out of the body is also a potent and powerful energy. In yogic traditions, the breath is called *prana,* or life force, the powerful current of energy that animates and enlivens us. The practice of consciously manipulating the breath is pranayama—*ayama* translates to "regulate." When you do a pranayama exercise, you are tapping into a tried-and-true methodology. Ancient yoga practitioners discovered that specific breathing techniques could improve health and well-being while calming and clearing the mind, and the system still stands today. This practice is old!

Pranayama exercises can improve mental focus and help you get more restorative, restful sleep each night. Luckily, you don't need to be a yogi or even spiritually minded to experience the power of the breath. While pranayama is a vast and intricate discipline, with over 50 different exercises listed in the Vedas, the ancient Sanskrit text that outlines yogic practice and philosophy, experimenting with just one consistently is all it takes to tap into the benefits of the practice.

Once you get comfortable using the breath as a tool—don't worry, I'll show you how— you can use it to prepare for a big presentation or a first date, to ready yourself for sleep, or to give yourself a jolt when feeling groggy. And the more comfortable you get with using the breath to calm and center the mind, the easier it will be to use your breathing to work for you in other ways, too. The breath is a path to feeling more calm and confident. In my yoga classes, I guide students through the process of harnessing the breath to release

Alternate Nostril Breathing: Nadi Shodhana

Nadi Shodhana is a powerful form of pranayama. By bringing focused attention to both nostrils, the practice is said to synchronize the two hemispheres of the brain (connecting our emotional side to our logical side), strengthen the respiratory system, and balance the nervous system. We tend to favor one nostril over the other, and Nadi Shodhana encourages an equal distribution of oxygen to each side of the brain—the left nostril represents the right side of the brain and the right nostril connects to the left—perking up cognitive function considerably.

Just 2 minutes of this pranayama can bring about notable effects. And a modified version of alternate nostril breathing can be a wonderful way to wind down. If you have trouble falling asleep, you can practice this pose in bed by lying on your right side and closing your right nostril with your right thumb. Breathing slowly and deeply through your left nostril will activate the parasympathetic nervous system, which calms and relaxes the body and mind.

Find a comfortable seated position and breathe normally for a few moments. Lift your left hand, place your index finger and middle finger at the eyebrow center, and close your left nostril with your thumb.

Breathe through your right nostril for three counts. Close your right nostril with your ring finger, hold for a count, and then release your left nostril and exhale. Inhale through your left nostril for three counts, close your left nostril, hold for a count, and exhale through your right nostril. Repeat for eight rounds of breath.

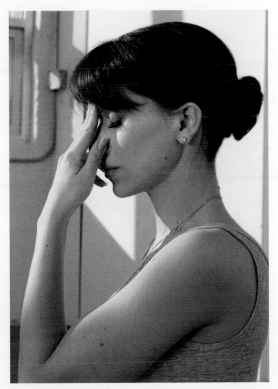

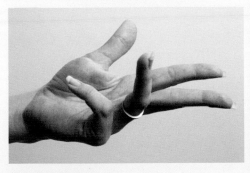

Hand Position

Sighs, Yawns, and Panting: Natural Ways the Body Uses the Breath

As you're paying more attention to the way you breathe, and how mindful breathing can change the way you feel, it can be helpful to note the clever techniques the body already has in place to calm the emotions and seek out more oxygen. Think of a sigh. We usually sigh when we're feeling frustrated or blue, but there's a physiological motivation behind the action. Scientists believe that sighing allows the air sacs in the lungs to relax, which acts as a reset for the entire respiratory system. If our breathing is disrupted by a stressful situation, sighing can be an especially effective way to resume a normal breath pattern, and calm, regulated breathing brings emotional relief. Yawning is another way the body takes breathing matters into its own hands. It's not entirely clear why we yawn, but we seem to do it when we're sleepy or stressed or when we see someone else yawning—it's contagious! Some researchers say we yawn because the brain needs more oxygen, but more recent studies point to thermoregulation—yawning may help cool the brain. Our sleep cycles and our stress cycles are linked to changes in brain temperature. We yawn just after temperatures rise, and things cool down up there after yawning. And if you find yourself panting (ideally this happens only while doing strenuous exercise), that's your body's way of seeking more oxygen. As you exercise more regularly, your body's capacity to extract oxygen from the blood will increase and panting will decrease.

tightness and tension in the body. The instruction to "breathe into your hamstrings" may sound strange (your lungs are not in your legs, right?). But it's a simple and effective visualization exercise that sends softening and opening energy to the spot in the body where you are placing your breathing attention.

Try it now! Move into a pose that is challenging for you, perhaps Forward Bend if your hamstrings are tight or Pigeon Pose if your hips are tight, and when you hit your edge, that place where you don't feel like you can go any further without injuring yourself, stop there and breathe. Take deep, controlled breaths and imagine the place that's tight gently opening and releasing. With each breath, send easeful, softening energy to the point of tension. Breathe for five counts (an inhalation and exhalation is one count), and then slowly move out of the pose. Take a few breaths and feel the results of your practice. Notice how exhalation has helped to release tension from the body. If you are in a pose that has two sides, like Pigeon, take a moment to note how the side you've yet to work on differs from the side that just received all that juicy breathing energy. Then move into the second side.

I often find that my private students are amazing mirrors for me. They usually come to me with an issue that I have tackled in my own life, so I really understood where Susanna was coming from when her challenges began to reveal themselves to me. She came to me in hopes of "perfecting her yoga practice," but within our lessons, I saw how her obsession with perfection was seeping into every aspect of her life, leaving her perpetually dissatisfied—with herself and others—and deeply unhappy. This played out on her mat. If she wobbled or fell while taking on challenging poses, a totally natural and expected part of the practice, she would take it very hard, sighing loudly and making excuses, like she was tired from a long day at the office and so on. Sometimes she would even get frustrated with me, telling me my routines did not have smooth transitions or that I wasn't clear enough in my instruction. After a few months of working with Susanna, I told her that breath work would be the focus of our practice that evening. She rolled her eyes in exasperation, a look I'd seen on students' faces many times when preparing them to work with the breath. I knew what Susanna was thinking (it's what most type A fitness folks think): the breath has nothing to do with getting their bodies in shape, that breathing is easy and obvious. I told her not to worry, that I'd still kick her butt, and I slowly walked her through a challenging sequence. Every time she wobbled in a standing pose, I would ask her to use the breath to find balance. Instead of letting her get frustrated and hold her breath (what we do when we're frustrated), I would encourage her to take long, deep breaths with exaggerated exhalations. She was so wrapped up in breathing and feeling her body in each pose that she forgot to be hard on herself, or me. We did this kind of work for a few more sessions, and I started to notice changes in her demeanor; she seemed to be lightening up—on me and herself!

Soon after, I sat her down and told her what I was doing. I let her know that I had noted her behavior toward me at the beginning of our time together and that I could see improvement after just a few weeks of working with the breath. Becoming familiar with

> I often find that my private students are amazing mirrors for me.

The Simple Art of Vinyasa: Linking Breath to Movement

The breath is the bridge between the body and the mind. When you bring your attention to your breathing, you quiet the noisy thinking of the mind and link it to what the body is doing at that very moment. As a result, you click back into the present, and away from fear and anxiety, and you also give the body the undivided attention it deserves, tuning in to what's really happening in your physical experience. You can tap into this mind-body connection in seated meditation, but you can also experience it while moving. Vinyasa, or flow yoga, is a style of yoga that links each movement to a breath. This is my favorite way to practice yoga since it is vigorous, energizing, and meditative all at once. I have created special vinyasa sequences for each of the Five Principles (at the end of each principle chapter), but you can get a taste of the melding of mind and body with this mini vinyasa flow that can be practiced at any time. I will do this mini flow while waiting for something to cook, before walking out the door, or while watching a movie.

A MINI YOGA FLOW:
ONE BREATH, ONE MOVEMENT

Start in Mountain Pose at the top of your mat. Inhale your arms up, exhale Forward Fold, inhale Half Lift, exhale Forward Fold, inhale Plank Pose, exhale Chaturanga, inhale Upward Facing Dog, exhale Downward Facing Dog, inhale your right leg to Downward Facing Dog Split, exhale step your foot between your hands and spiral the back heel down to the mat, inhale Warrior 1, exhale Warrior 2, inhale Peaceful Warrior, exhale Chaturanga, inhale Upward Dog, exhale Downward Facing Dog. Repeat on your left side.

her breath and using it consciously was helping her to navigate through her frustration. At this point, Susanna opened up to me, letting me know that she walked through most of her life irritated and angry with herself and the world. She never felt like she was doing a good enough job, and as a result, she often wasn't; she wasn't using her time wisely, and she felt inefficient, overwhelmed, and anxious at work and in her personal life. And she wasn't having fun. She was finally ready to admit that she didn't want to live this way anymore.

From that moment on, she was aware of her challenges and had some tools to tackle them. She would bring her attention to her breath when she felt stress creeping up, taking a few minutes to consciously count her inhalations and exhalations before returning to her work. This was really exciting to see, but I was careful to remind her that yoga and Living Clearly are lifelong practices, not a perfection. They're not about mastery of a specific breathing exercise or a particular pose. They're about integrating these ways into your everyday life, turning to them as tools and resources along the way.

Breathing may be considered the most important of all of the functions of the body, for, indeed, all the other functions depend upon it. Man may exist some time without eating; a shorter time without drinking; but without breathing his existence may be measured by a few minutes. And not only is Man dependent upon Breath for life, but he is largely dependent upon correct habits of breathing for continued vitality and freedom from disease. An intelligent control of our breathing power will lengthen our days upon earth by giving us increased vitality and powers of resistance, and, on the other hand, unintelligent and careless breathing will tend to shorten our days, by decreasing our vitality and laying us open to disease.

—YOGI RAMACHARAKA, *SCIENCE OF BREATH*

BREATHING THROUGH STRESSFUL SITUATIONS

Starting today, begin to track the way you breathe, paying specific attention to the situations and emotions that change your breathing patterns. Like an inspired researcher, record your findings in a journal. Note the moments where your breathing gets short and shallow, and see what happens if you bring your focus to your breath and if you consciously change the way you're breathing, practicing one of the exercises in this chapter or simply regulating your inhalations and exhalations so they are smooth and steady. Notice where your breath gets sacrificed, the moments in your life when you give it up instantaneously. See what happens when you decide—remember, it's all a choice—to slow yourself down with a few conscious breaths, breathing in for a few counts and then extending the exhale a bit longer. Can you start to use the breath to calm your nervous system, to create spaciousness where there was once claustrophobic reactivity? Jot it all down in a journal for a week, and then review your findings. You may be surprised.

If all this breathing talk still seems out there, there are some concrete places to start. Here are some of the most common ways we lose the breath. The next time you encounter one of these circumstances or emotions, notice what your breath is up to and then experiment with mindful breathing before reacting. There is a very good chance that the course of action you commit to after breathing will be quite different from the one you would have pursued without the breath. Note your findings.

LATENESS. Notice when you are late for work, school, or an appointment. What happens to your breath? Can you slow it down? Can you breathe deeper? Can you relax the tensed muscles taking over your body (think: jaw, shoulders, neck, brow)? Remember, getting stressed won't get you there any faster. Is all the tension and pain worth it?

FRUSTRATION. What happens to your breath when the waiter doesn't get your order right even though you told him three times? Where does your breath go when your roommate leaves her dishes in the sink—again? What about when your teenager forgets to clean his room—again? Notice what is happening to your body in these situations. Stop. Take a few calming breaths. Once your breathing is steady, you are ready to respond.

FEAR. Are you afraid of flying, public speaking, rejection, intimacy? Each one must be met with a calm and steady breath. Withholding the breath will only make the situation worse, causing your heart to beat faster and your body to contract and freeze up. If you

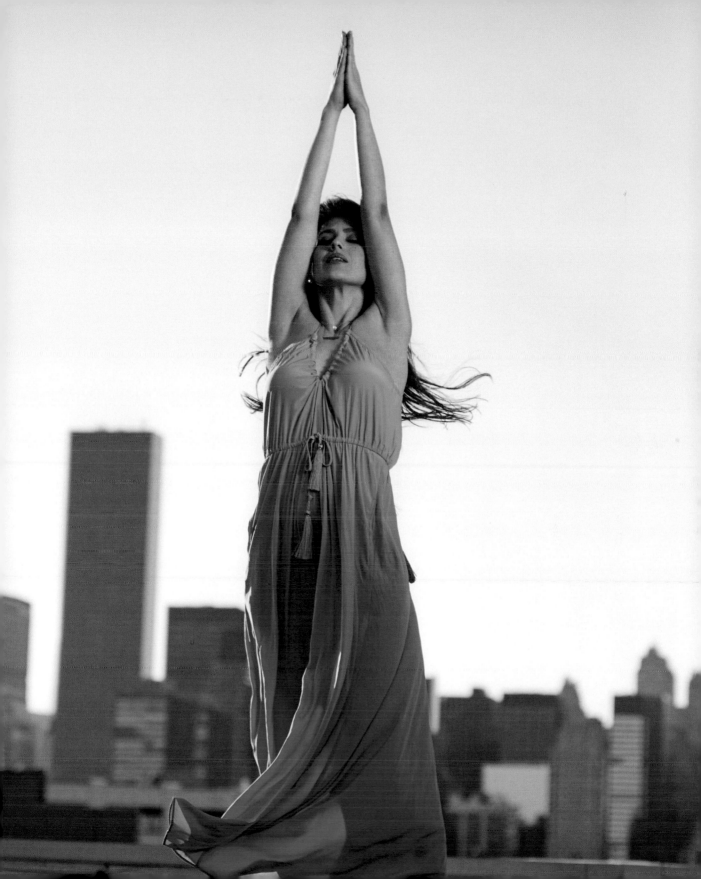

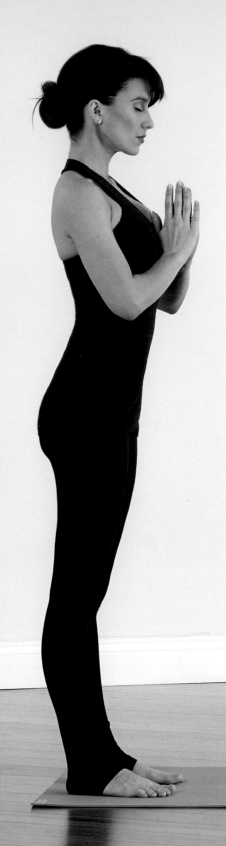

Mountain Pose: Tadasana

Mountain Pose, or Tadasana, is a foundational yoga posture, the starting point for almost all yoga sequences and the place to which you return throughout your practice. Though it looks simple—you're just standing there, right?—it's filled with opportunities to strengthen your foundation, to feel your muscular and skeletal systems working together harmoniously, and to activate the power of the breath. Tadasana is a great place to feel your breath moving up and down your body, elongating your spine with each inhalation. You can experiment with different visualizations, imagining your breath moving up the back of your body, following your spine up into the crown of your head, and then moving down the front of your body all the way through your legs and feet and into the ground. Just as you practiced using the breath to release tension and tightness in the body, you can also use the breath to create more space in the body, to elongate and open. See yourself getting taller with each breath—be sure to keep all four corners of your feet on the ground (I'll talk about the empowering process of grounding in the next chapter)—and rooting into the earth.

To move into Tadasana, simply stand with your feet together and your toes and heels touching. Lift up all 10 toes, spread them, and then gently relax them down on the floor. Pull up through your arches and zip up through your legs, feeling the activation of your inner thighs toward one another. Activate your quads, pulling your knees up into them, feeling your legs long and strong. Take one hand to your belly and one to the base of your back. Activate your navel in toward your spine, lengthening your lumbar (lower) spine. Relax your glutes and feel your tailbone releasing down toward the ground. Take your hands to the bottom of your rib cage, feel that you are bringing them into your body, opening up the back and creating space in between your shoulder blades for your thoracic spine. Bring your hands to prayer, tuck your chin slightly, and feel the back of your neck lengthening, reaching the crown of your head toward the ceiling. Imagine your spine like a bungee cord, lengthening in two directions—down and up. Release your shoulder blades down your back.

are afraid to fly, practice deep and rhythmic breathing continuously before your trip. When you board the plane, take your seat, close your eyes, and practice Sama Vritti breathing. The chances of a disaster are minuscule, but your panic wouldn't stop one from happening anyway. Use the breath to quiet your racing mind; notice how the dark scenarios begin to fade away as you bring yourself into the present moment with your breath. If you have to speak in front of a group, prepare thoroughly so you are ready to share your thoughts, and then practice your breathing before getting onstage. Entering the moment in an already calm state is key to maintaining composure and giving your brilliant content the chance to be heard clearly by your audience.

RAGE. Anger has a particularly volatile relationship with the breath. When you get enraged, you are overcome with the emotion; it's as if a dark, sticky ooze creeps up all over you until you are dominated by the angry feelings. And the breath is the first to go. There is no room for calm, steady breathing when you are filled with rage. As a first step, I recommend removing yourself from the situation. This may look like moving into another room or taking a short walk. You have gained perspective when you can zoom out enough to imagine how you'd feel if you had succumbed to the tantalizing pull of your emotions, saying something you would regret later. Often, simply creating some physical distance between you and the conflict is enough to kick-start your zooming-out mechanism.

Breathing is your ticket to a peaceful mind and a happy heart. It will guide you to the best of you, that place where you can make wise decisions unburdened by reactivity. And mindful breathing is the bridge between the body and the mind, a surefire way to quiet mental chatter and listen closely to what the body has to say. Simply bringing your attention to the air as it moves through your nasal passages and feeling your ribs and belly expanding with each breath click your mind into your body's experience and into the freedom of the present moment. From here you begin to really feel yourself in the heart of your life, standing firmly on the earth, cultivating the sense of belonging that we all deserve. And now you're ready to experience the stabilizing influence of grounding. Onward!

YOGA FOR BREATHING

Yoga asanas and breathing are intimately connected; you can't have one without the other. Any yoga pose you move into will involve the breath, but you can bring specific awareness to how you're breathing while you transition in and out of poses, focusing on connecting an inhalation or exhalation to each movement. As you inhale, feel your rib cage expand, and as you exhale, feel your body soften. Notice the poses where breathing is more challenging and those where it is expansive and open. Welcoming your breath into your practice like this brings a vitality and dynamism to every moment on your mat. *Note:* This sequence opens with **SAMA VRITTI,** a simple but powerful breathing exercise. *Approximately 10 minutes*

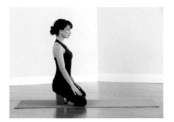

❶ Come to a comfortable seated position. Close your eyes, and bring your attention to your breath. You are looking for an inhalation and exhalation that are equal in length. Inhale through your nose, and then exhale through your nose a few times. Now, inhale through your nose and exhale out your mouth like you are fogging a mirror. This sound should have a deep oceanic quality. Notice how that changes the feeling of your breath. Again, inhale nose, exhale mouth. Close your lips, inhale through your nose, and exhale out your nose, maintaining that same oceanic sound with your breath in the back of your throat. It's common to get a little lightheaded with this practice, so take a break or close your eyes if you feel dizzy. You can also do this exercise lying down. Now, inhale through your nose for one count and exhale out for one count. Inhale one, exhale one. Now, inhale one, two. Hold your breath in for a moment, and then exhale for one, two. Hold your breath out for a moment. Inhale one, two. Hold. Exhale one, two. Hold. Now, inhale one, two, three. Hold. Exhale one, two, three. Hold. Inhale one, two, three. Hold. Exhale one, two, three. Hold. Inhale one, two, three, four. Hold. Exhale one, two, three, four. Hold. Inhale one, two, three, four. Hold. Exhale one, two, three, four. Hold. Make sure you are not speeding up the counts! Inhale one, two, three, four, five. Hold. Exhale one, two, three, four, five. Hold. Inhale one, two, three, four, five. Hold. Exhale one, two, three, four, five. Hold. Inhale one, two, three, four, five, six. Hold. Exhale one, two, three, four, five, six. Hold. Inhale one, two, three, four, five, six. Hold. Exhale one, two, three, four, five, six. Hold. Now, breathe normally, and while inhaling and exhaling, notice how much more we focus on the inhale than the exhale. But you don't want to throw that part of the breath away! You can create a longer breath by drawing the breath in at a slower rate and letting it out at a slower rate. This is also an excellent way to increase the capacity of your lungs. This oceanic breath—in through the nose, out through the nose—is called *ujjayi* breathing. It is an invigorating breath that will not only work your lungs but will also heat your body up from the inside out. Keep the Sama Vritti evenness to your breath, trying to not hold it throughout your practice. Your breath is vital to your health and life. So focus on it, make it a priority, and notice all the good things that will come from your effort.

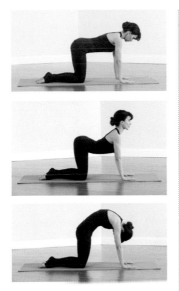

② Transition onto all fours and move into **CAT COW**. Spread your fingers wide, and shift your weight from side to side. Inhale, arch your back, and look up into **COW** pose. Exhale, press into your hands and knees, draw your navel toward your back, round your spine, and look down into **CAT** pose. Inhale arch, exhale round. Take three full rounds of *ujjayi* breath, matching the movements to each inhale and exhale.

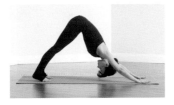

③ Come to a neutral spine, walk your knees back a few inches, exhale and curl your toes under, and take your hips high and your heels low into **DOWNWARD FACING DOG**. Take a moment to warm up your body: Peddle your feet and sway your hips from side to side. Bend one knee deeply and then the other, and let your head hang heavy on your neck. Then clean up your **DOWNWARD FACING DOG**: Make sure your hands are shoulder-width apart and your feet are hip-distance apart. Spread your fingers and toes. Press the floor away with your hands and ground down with your heels. Feel your spine lengthening. There should be no tension in your neck. Take three rounds of breath, each time thinking about creating space between the muscles and bones of your body.

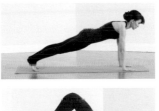

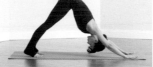

④ Inhale slowly into **PLANK POSE**, and then exhale slowly back into **DOWNWARD FACING DOG**. Take three rounds of complete breath here, transitioning between **PLANK** and **DOWNWARD FACING DOG** with each inhale and exhale.

Sun Salutation A

Match a breath to each movement in this sequence.

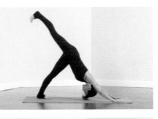

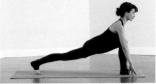

⑤ Inhale your right leg up. Exhale step your right foot through your hands into **LOW LUNGE**. Inhale, open up your chest, and extend long through your back leg.

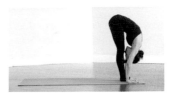

⑥ Exhale step your left foot to meet your right at the front of your mat. Your head hangs heavy in **UTTANASANA** (aka Forward Fold).

(continued)

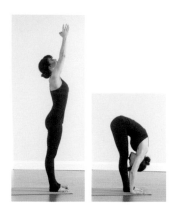

7 Inhale reach your arms up into **MOUNTAIN POSE**.

8 Exhale, hands come through your center as you fold all the way down into a deep **FORWARD BEND/FOLD/UTTANASANA**.

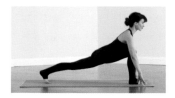

9 Inhale step your right leg back into **LOW LUNGE**.

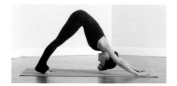

10 Exhale **DOWNWARD FACING DOG**.

11 Inhale transition your shoulders forward into **PLANK POSE**, keeping your heels reaching toward the back of your mat.

12 Exhale lower down to **KNEES**, **CHEST**, **CHIN**, arching your back strongly.

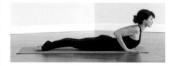

13 Inhale draw yourself forward into **BABY COBRA**, squeezing your shoulder blades, activating your elbows toward one another, and pressing your palms into the floor right beside your lower rib cage.

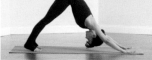

14 Exhale press away through **CHILD'S POSE** into **DOWNWARD FACING DOG**.

15 Inhale your shoulders forward into **PLANK**.

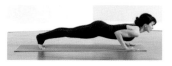

16 Exhale **CHATURANGA** (modify by lowering down to your knees if that is appropriate for you).

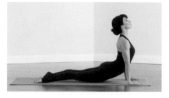

17 Inhale **UPWARD FACING DOG**, your knees off the floor. (Don't lose the breath as the sequence gets more challenging.)

18 Exhale **DOWNWARD FACING DOG**.

Repeat on your left side, ending in Downward Facing Dog.

Sun Salutation B

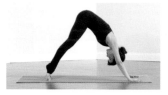

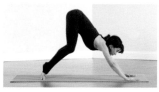

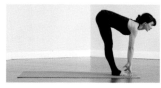

1 Inhale tippy toes. Exhale, bend your knees, and look forward. Inhale jump or step to the front of your mat, finishing in **HALF LIFT**.

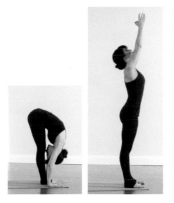

2 Exhale **FORWARD BEND**.

3 Inhale **MOUNTAIN POSE**.

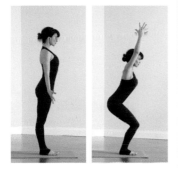

4 Exhale stand up tall with your hands by your sides.

5 Inhale sit down into **CHAIR POSE**.

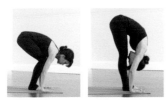

6 Exhale touch the floor with your hands, and then straighten your knees into **FORWARD FOLD**.

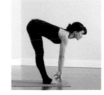

7 Inhale **HALF LIFT**.

8 Exhale jump or step back into **CHATURANGA**.

9 Inhale **UPWARD DOG**.

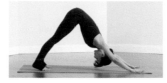

10 Exhale **DOWNWARD FACING DOG**, grounding your heels with your sit bones high.

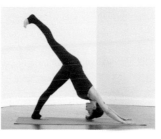

11 Inhale your right leg up, squaring your hips.

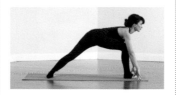

12 Exhale bring your foot between your hands, spiraling your back heel down to your mat at a 45-degree angle.

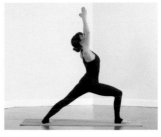

13 Inhale rise up to **WARRIOR 1**, with your arms raised above your head, your front knee over your ankle, and the outer edge of your back foot firmly sealed into the floor. Rotate your left hip toward the front of your mat, maintaining a strong, straight back leg.

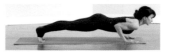

14 Exhale your hands to the floor on either side of your front foot moving into **CHATURANGA**. This feels like a fast transition with one breath, but it gets easier with practice! The more you breathe, the greater your lung capacity will be.

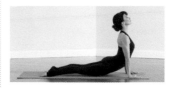

15 Inhale **UPWARD DOG**.

16 Exhale **DOWNWARD FACING DOG**.

Repeat on your left side, ending in Downward Facing Dog.

(continued)

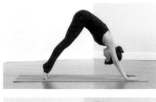

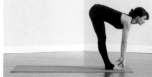

1 Inhale tippy toes. Exhale, bend your knees, and look forward. Inhale jump or step to the front of your mat, finishing in **HALF LIFT**.

2 Exhale **FORWARD BEND**.

3 Inhale **MOUNTAIN POSE**.

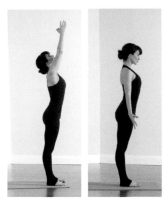

4 Exhale release your hands by your sides.

5 Inhale sit into **CHAIR POSE**.

6 Exhale your hands to the floor and then straighten your legs **FORWARD FOLD**.

7 Inhale **HALF LIFT**.

8 Exhale **CHATURANGA**.

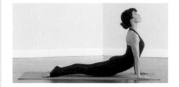

9 Inhale **UPWARD DOG**.

10 Exhale **DOWNWARD FACING DOG**.

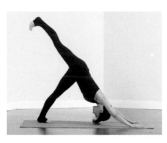

11 Inhale lift your right leg.

12 Exhale place the foot in between your hands, spiraling the back heel down to the mat at a 45-degree angle.

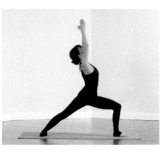

13 Inhale lift your arms up into **WARRIOR 1**.

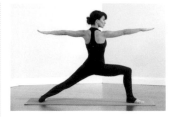

14 Exhale open your right arm forward and your left arm back into **WARRIOR 2**. Your knee should be directly over your ankle, your shoulders soft, and your arms expanding. Your rib cage and pelvis should be perfectly stacked. Use your core to lengthen your spine. Gaze over your right fingertips, which should be active and aware.

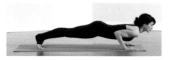

15 Inhale frame your front foot with your hands, and then exhale into **CHATURANGA**.

16 Inhale **UPWARD DOG**, keeping your arms strong and your legs off the floor.

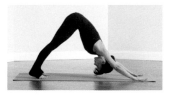

17 Exhale **DOWNWARD FACING DOG**.

Repeat on your left side, ending in Downward Facing Dog.

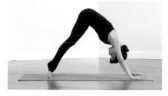

1 Inhale tippy toes. Exhale, bend your knees, and look forward. Inhale jump or step to the front of your mat, finishing in **HALF LIFT**.

2 Exhale **FORWARD BEND**.

3 Inhale **MOUNTAIN POSE**.

4 Exhale release your hands by your sides.

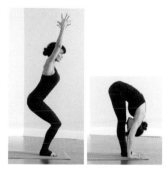

5 Inhale sit down into **CHAIR POSE**.

6 Exhale **FORWARD BEND**.

7 Inhale **HALF LIFT**.

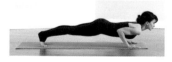

8 Exhale **CHATURANGA**.

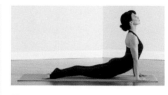

9 Inhale **UPWARD DOG**.

10 Exhale **DOWNWARD FACING DOG**.

11 Inhale lift your right leg up.

12 Exhale step your foot between your hands, spiraling your back heel down to your mat at a 45-degree angle.

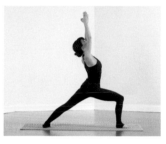

13 Inhale **WARRIOR 1**, squaring off your hips.

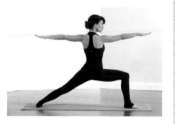

14 Exhale open your arms into **WARRIOR 2**.

15 Inhale, tip back, releasing your left hand down your left leg, reaching your right arm

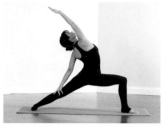

up and over your head into **PEACEFUL WARRIOR**.

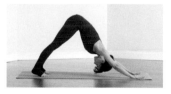

16 Exhale windmill your hands to the floor and lowering through **CHATURANGA**.

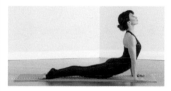

17 Inhale **UPWARD DOG**.

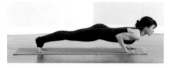

18 Exhale **DOWNWARD FACING DOG**.

Repeat on your left side.

Come to a seated position, allowing yourself to resume a regular breath. Note the exercised breath and the sensations you feel throughout your body.

To be rooted is perhaps the most important and least recognized need of the human soul.

—SIMONE WEIL

Chapter Six

THE THIRD PRINCIPLE

GROUNDING

YOUR LIST OF THINGS TO ACCOMPLISH TODAY IS LONG AND WINDING: things to do at work and things to do at home, administrative tasks and intellectually challenging projects. People are counting on you to get things done. The phone's ringing, e-mail's popping, baby's crying, and you're starting to come undone. Your brain feels fuzzy, your vision is blurry, and you seem to have floated a million miles away. It's practically an out-of-body experience. But instead of taking a moment to regroup, you push harder, reaching for another coffee or a sugary treat or just muscling through all you have to do.

For most of us, this is just an average day navigating the terrain of our nonstop modern society. Whether you're a stay-at-home mom, a high-powered executive, or a combination of the two, there is no escaping the incessant beat of this drum. You may be a single yoga teacher in Miami or a married writer in Toledo; it doesn't matter. Unless you live off the grid and do nothing but grow your own food—which has its own unique kind of pressure, too—you are sucked, daily, into the buzzy, busy pace of today's world. Most of us are walking around in a daze of multitasking freneticism, tapping away at our not-so-smart phones while walking, driving (please, no!), buying groceries, and running on the treadmill. We eat dinner standing up, we watch TV while taking a shower, and we rock our babies while we swipe away on our phones. Technology makes us hyperconnected and overly available. When we're not vigilant, we gorge on social media, filling our brains with sparkling images of happy, beautiful strangers or friends of friends. Then we inflate the images with assumption and speculation, believing that everyone else is happier, healthier, and having more fun than we are.

Our plates are filled to overflowing; it's as if we're at an all-you-can-eat buffet of things that must get done, and we don't know how to put down our forks. With this much stimulation coming at us 24/7, feeling overwhelmed has become our current affliction. And being overwhelmed is the gateway drug to more serious emotional challenges. Experience it too often, and you'll soon find yourself depressed, anxious, sad, and afraid.

> Grounding is the antidote to being overwhelmed.

We're looking for a burst of control in a life that seems to have none. Instead of turning toward the body, using it as a refuge in a reality that has become overwhelming, we work to escape it with extreme behavior and harmful habits. We check out, but the only way to change things is to check in, to sink deeper into the body.

Moving from perspective to breathing delivers you ripe and ready for the next of the Living Clearly Principles, grounding. The breath carried you from the mind to the body, bringing you into a felt sense of what's happening in your physical being right this very minute (if you need a refresher, try any of the breathing exercises in Chapter Five). And now, here, settled in the body, you can deepen your experience of Living Clearly and get even more access to the wisdom and information held within by bringing your focus to grounding. It's a very simple and practical principle. We are swept away by our thoughts so often that we lose touch with our own form; we forget that our feet are always connected to the ground.

I like to imagine grounding like the foundation of my house. If the foundation is shaky, my home will be unstable; the first big gust of wind that blows through will send it spinning out into Oz. But if my foundation is rock solid, no inclement weather will be able to touch it. Same goes for life. When we are grounded, we can easily gather ourselves when we're feeling anxious, fragmented, scattered, or overwhelmed. In fact, grounding is the antidote to being overwhelmed. That panicky, disconnected, out-of-body feeling doesn't stand a chance when you can feel your feet on the ground, or your butt on your chair, and

TAKE A TECH BREAK

Turn off your phone, close the computer, and take a break from technology. You hear it all the time, but can you actually step away for a moment? Our gadgets have become our lifelines, and there's a sense that the earth might actually stop spinning or something awful might happen if we put them down. But a time-out from connectivity can be the ultimate in self-care, a clear message to yourself and the world that you need some healthy space. I have a friend who runs her own business. To keep herself from working nonstop, she forces herself to step away from her computer for the entire weekend. She tells her clients at the outset that she doesn't work on weekends; if you e-mail her on Saturday or Sunday, you will receive an automatic message that says she'll be back online early Monday and will respond to you then.

If zero computer time is too intense, or impossible, you can give yourself a mini social media cleanse. I like cleanses more than fasts, because I believe that we all need to consume to stay alive. Just like a cleanse where you cut out foods that are irritants and allergens—like wheat, dairy, and so on—you can stop or limit your social media usage for a day, a week, a month, or longer. If you are a heavy user, start with a day. Taking a break will show you just how much time you spend with your face turned toward a screen. Imagine what you can do with all of that found time!

when you can root down and experience the sensation of your body on the earth. When you can tap into grounding, challenging situations will not have the power to rock you.

When we activate grounding, we tap into our own personal source of safety and security, two elements that must be in place for us to be able to reach a desired outcome. How can you pursue a professional goal, dive into a love relationship, or reach a fitness milestone if you don't feel safe? Since life is inherently unpredictable and uncertain and the only thing we can really count on is change itself, the ability to click into a true sense of grounding becomes a lifeline.

The body is your source of grounding. We spend so much time wrapped up in the fluctuations and demands of our minds, getting sucked into complex thoughts, theories, ideas, and imaginings, searching desperately for answers and solutions, that we forget that all the guidance we need is already with us, *is us*. The body is inherently simple and clear-cut, and when we ground, we have access to its knowledge, which can guide us

(continued on page 80)

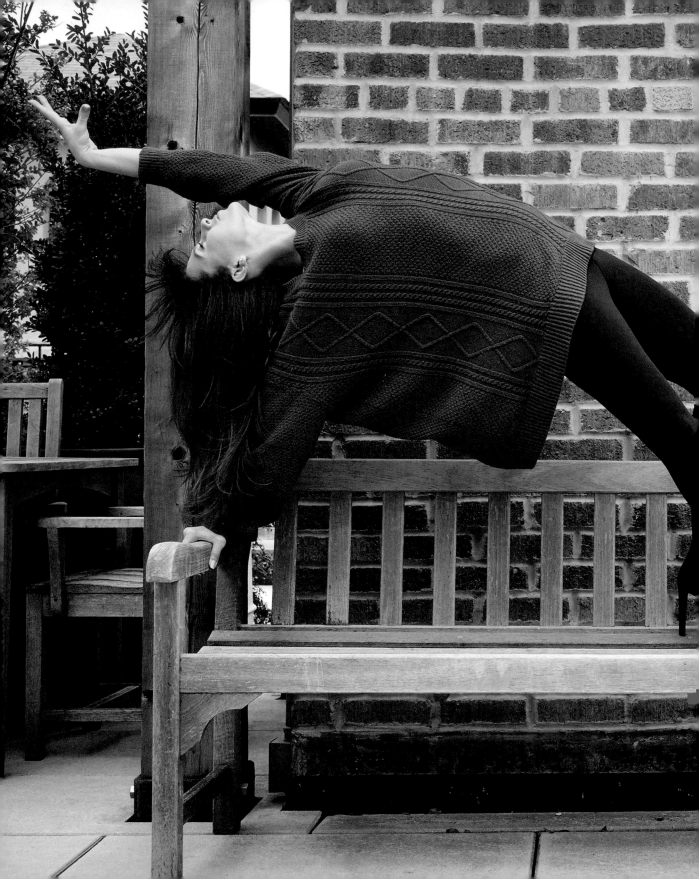

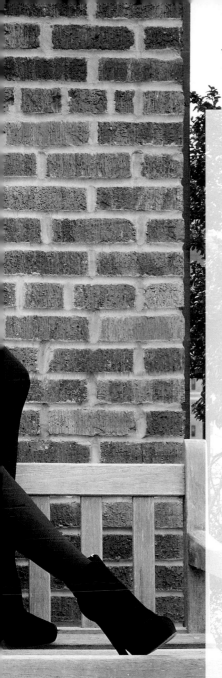

An Everyday Grounding Practice

Like perspective and breathing, grounding can be practiced anywhere, at any moment in your life. You don't need to do a specific exercise—though the exercises in this chapter and the Yoga for Grounding sequence at the end of this chapter are excellent ways to cultivate grounding muscle memory, making it even easier to click into the practice when you need it most. You may be rolling around on the carpet with your toddler, walking down the street, standing in line, driving your car (driving is an excellent laboratory for experimentation with the Living Clearly Principles because we are often challenged when behind the wheel!), in a meeting with a huge client, negotiating a raise with your boss, or in a difficult conversation with your partner. Whatever the circumstance, it is guaranteed that a good part of your body will be in contact with the surface that is holding it up, which means you can practice grounding.

Try it now. Wherever you are this very moment—on the subway, in bed, leaning on a counter or against a wall—is the perfect place to practice grounding. Feel your body wherever it is making contact with the surface that's holding it up. If you are in bed, feel the bed holding you firmly and completely. You are safe and held. If you are sitting, notice your sit bones as they rest against the chair or your seat on the train, bus, or car. Feel your foundation strong and stable. If you are standing, sense your feet in your socks and your socks in your shoes and feel those shoes upon the ground. Imagine the depth of the earth that is supporting you. Like a tall oak tree, your roots go deep and your branches go high. You are strong, stable, capable, and wise.

When we ground, we become deeply at home in ourselves. We start to believe that we actually belong here and that what we have to offer is legitimate and wonderful because we feel supported. A regular grounding practice—you can ground all day if you want to!—helps you feel calm and safe, and from there, you can connect to the part of yourself that is clear and wise, the part that would give commonsense advice to an anxious friend.

through anything. Whether you're at a fork in the road, called to make a decision that will change the course of your life (take that job in another country, marry that person who's ready to commit to you, start a family), or just looking for an easier way to get through each day, grounding helps you connect to the essence of who you are, which sets you up to find balance (see Chapter Seven), the place from which you can make good decisions.

You could be on the 45th floor of an urban office building, feeling rocked by a conflict you just had with your boss or a colleague, but you can still pull back to gain perspective, take a couple of mindful breaths, and then begin to feel your body in the chair you're sitting in, sense that chair on the floor, know that the floor is part of the building, and the building is standing steady on the earth. When you tap into that connected force, really feeling the depth and sturdiness of your foundation, you will begin to see that doubt, insecurity, anxiety, fear, and worry start to vaporize from your body, and you have access to a knowing that will help you make your next move. Unexpected obstacles will always be part of your life, but when you cultivate the ability to ground in any situation, you will be able to deftly navigate life's obstacle course.

Over the past few years, I've had several opportunities to practice grounding in my own life. Each of these challenging moments threatened to sweep my feet out from under me and completely rock my universe, but with a conscious activation of grounding energies (in tandem with the other Living Clearly Principles), I always managed to call back the pieces of my fragmented self and feel whole again. And the more I practice, the easier it gets! I'm at the point now where I can usually calm my racing heart or jagged nerve endings quite quickly, and then I'm on my toes again, ready for anything life has to give me. Let me be clear, this does not mean that I never feel my foundation rumble or that I don't experience huge waves of emotion. Oh, I do. But while things are happening and the feelings are rolling over me in big messy waves, I can grasp onto a lifeline and find a way to pull myself back to shore.

This happened a few years ago at a high-profile event in NYC. I was asked to be the master of ceremonies for a youth dance performance at Lincoln Center in Manhattan. I've performed since I was 2, so stage fright has never been a part of my life, but this night was different. I had assumed that I would be greeted by a knowledgeable point person and walked through the program and what was expected of me that evening, but when I arrived backstage, I was met by someone who was clearly unfamiliar with the event and my role in it all. He brusquely walked me through a few disconnected talking points and

Exercise: Building a Sense of Grounding

When I work one-on-one with clients who are struggling with low self-esteem or who can't see the beauty in themselves at any level, I give them this homework assignment. It's a simple exercise that anyone can do, but the results can be extraordinary when practiced regularly.

1. Stand with your feet hip-width apart. (Hip width is only two fists wide and no more. You may think your hips are wider, but they're not. Trust me!) Feel your weight sinking into the ground. Flex and relax your toes. Keeping your feet in one place, shift your weight forward, back, and side to side. Feel all four corners of your feet come alive.

2. Take your hands to your hips and press down like you are making yourself heavier.

3. Repeat shifting and relaxing and flexing your feet. Bend and straighten your knees.

4. Try to jump from this position. Can you even make it off the ground? This is the sensation of being grounded—heavy, solid, and firm.

5. Now, bend your knees very low and jump up (even a tiny hop), feeling your weight spring up and then return to a grounded position when you reconnect with the earth. Feel your feet in contact with the floor and pull your strength up from there, like a volcano pulls its fire up from the center of the earth.

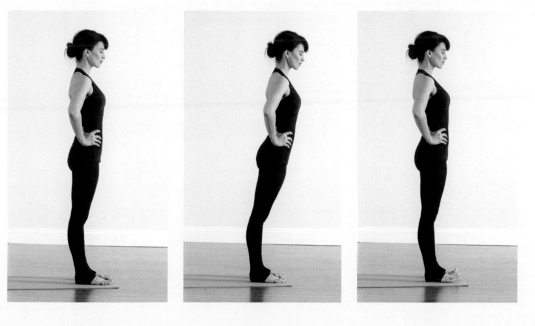

then began ripping typed paragraphs out of sheets of paper to reorganize and scrawl new notes with a Sharpie. My heart began to beat faster. I had been to enough events to know that hosting something of this size would require tight, clear notes delivered on a prompter. When I asked for clarification, he only furthered the ripping of pages and scrawling of new notes. It was all incredibly jumbled and disorganized, and I could feel myself starting to freak out. My head was spinning, my vision was getting blurry, and I felt as if I were floating off of the ground.

Here I was, at one of the country's most esteemed venues for the arts, with hundreds of people in the audience—and I had no idea what I was supposed to say. Before I knew it, I was in the center of the stage. I could feel the heat of the spotlight from there. I started shaking and felt incredibly small. I was so nervous and it was obvious. I began to stammer aloud and fumble through the mess that was my notes. I needed to pause, regroup, and ground myself. By pausing, I redirected the energy, which was hurtling toward paralyzing stage fright and a disastrous event. I zoomed out and was able to see that this evening didn't have to implode. I could save it (and myself!). I focused on my breathing and then turned my attention to grounding. There was a solution in here somewhere, but my mind was not going to find it. I breathed deeper and felt my muscles begin to relax. The tension in my head began to subside and now I could feel my feet. I sensed my feet in my shoes—stilettos, of course—and then every layer and strata beneath them, down into the core of the earth. Feeling into this multilayered foundation gave me strength. Now I was really beginning to see clearly and my common sense spoke up from within: *This is a dance performance and you are a dancer. You know what to do.*

> Grounding is not just a tool for getting through the shaky and unsure moments in life; new things are only possible if you can get unstuck.

Focusing on my voice, I asked for the basic information about the participants and the order of the performances. Then I walked out on the stage—no notes, no prompters. I knew that many of the people in the audience had come to watch their children perform, and I remembered how exciting it can be for the families of young dancers, so I said loudly and with a huge smile, "How many of you have a family member or loved one performing tonight?!" People started shouting proudly and clapping wildly. Even though I couldn't see their faces, this exchange helped me to connect with them and remember that we were all just people in a room together. I started to relax, and from there, the event unfolded more smoothly.

Even if you haven't been nose-to-nose with stage fright, you can tap into grounding anytime you feel nervous about speaking, like before a first date or a presentation at work or when preparing to have a significant conversation with someone you care about. Grounding neutralizes the uncertain and flighty feeling that comes from performance anxiety.

Grounding is not just a tool for getting through the shaky and unsure moments in life; new things are only possible if you can get unstuck, and grounding helps you do this by freeing you from the loop of defeating stories that can run nonstop in your head: *I'm not smart enough. I'm not pretty enough. I'm not skinny enough. She's doing it better than me. . . . I'm not smart enough. I'm not pretty enough. I'm not skinny enough. She's doing it better than me.* These stories are stagnant energy, delusional and untrue—and powerful. Until you bring attention to them, the dark tales you tell yourself live undisturbed, thriving and multiplying, infecting your life and your body like a virus.

And notice how you hold your body when you're insecure, unsure, or overwhelmed. Your head is likely hanging down and your shoulders hunched. This is a protective

FEEL YOUR FEET ON THE EARTH

We cannot fly, so our connection to the earth is so important. When was the last time your wiggled your bare toes in the grass or sunk your feet into a stream or the sand? If you live in a city, it might have been a long, long time ago. Getting grounded is about feeling yourself on the earth, and there's no better way do this than by getting your feet right into it. If you're an urban dweller, you can accomplish some toes-to-dirt connection without leaving town. Hit up your local park and get your feet naked. Run your toes through the grass, and dig them into the soil if you're daring. If you have the luxury of a backyard, take 5 minutes to get your feet on the earth every day. Getting barefoot is so simple. Try practicing any of the exercises in this chapter outside, or just take five to connect to the ground and stretch your arms up high. If you live in a chilly climate, strip off your socks at home. The important thing is to really feel your feet: When bare feet are pressed against a firm foundation, you become aware of the intricate complexity of bones, muscles, and tendons.

posture. Your body is responding to what your mind dictates (*I'm not fill-in-the-blank enough*), but you can break the cycle by using your physiology to call the shots. Stand tall and proud, feeling your feet connecting to the power of the earth, and you start to feel better about who you are. From there, you can access what you have to offer. You are deciding where you want your life to go. You are captured.

Take Amanda. She came to me for private lessons after her parents offered to help her get into better shape. Her family was wealthy, and though she had access to the best clothing and makeup, her self-confidence seemed to be quite low. She was overweight and had trouble maintaining eye contact. I wasn't sure private lessons were best for her; many people find that the collective experience of a group class helps to keep them motivated and intensifies their workout. But when she arrived at one of our meetings incredibly down and defeated, I knew that one-on-one work could really help her.

I asked her what was troubling her, and she showed me a photo of a super-handsome guy, tall and fit, with a nice jawline. They had been family friends for years, but she desperately longed to break out of the friend zone and explore something romantic. There was just one problem: She was convinced that she was not pretty enough to win this guy's affection. She burst into tears as she described herself as pimply and fat with frizzy hair. She said she was sweaty all the time and that her features were imperfect. She told me she didn't own a full-length mirror because she didn't want to see herself in her entirety. There was no mention of her infectious smile, bright eyes, and loving demeanor. It was clear that she had been running a negative story about herself for so many years that she was completely disconnected from who she really was. She was too much in her head—not enough on her feet.

We had some very real work to do together. My job was twofold. First, I acknowledged her concerns without blowing them off with a dismissive, "You are beautiful! Stop being so silly!" I wanted her to know that her experience was legitimate—even if her view of herself was distorted. We talked about ways to improve the appearance of her skin and hair and explored realistic ways of shifting her diet and exercising regularly. I connected her with a dermatologist and acupuncturist to help her with her skin and overall well-being, and I explained that if she were to eat healthier and get into better shape, her hormones would rebalance and she would stop sweating so profusely.

Next, I began the process of bringing her back into her body, so she could connect to who she really was and begin to have a different experience in her daily life. To do this,

Tadasana: Mountain Pose Part Two

You spent some time in Mountain Pose in the previous chapter, experiencing your breath as it moved up the back of your body and down the front. Now it's time to move deeper into this fundamental yoga pose by experiencing just how firmly your feet and legs can hold you up. You are strong and steady like the tallest mountain in the world. Your foundation can't be rocked, and your heights can't be summited. This pose can be practiced anywhere at any time. It is amazingly adaptable and a quick and easy way to reset and gather yourself before moving into any situation.

1. Move into Mountain Pose (see page 66 in Chapter Five for detailed directions).

2. Lift up all 10 toes and then softly place them back down. Picture yourself getting heavier and heavier, actively releasing into the floor, while continuing to lengthen the spine up. In our culture, we're so afraid of the word *heavy*, but heaviness is a good thing. It gives us a true sense of belonging on the earth, and it is the heart of grounding. Feel all of your body weight releasing through your feet into your mat. Feeling your substance is simply feeling yourself. With every inhale, focus on expanding your rib cage. With every exhale, allow tension to release from your body. Imagine that you are a tall and sturdy mountain. Your base is rock solid. You are massive, unshakable, earthy, and eternal.

we worked on grounding. As I walked her through vinyasa flows, I would consistently bring her back to the places where her body was touching the floor or making contact with itself. Sometimes her feet would be rooting into the floor as she reached up into a strong Mountain Pose. Other times, it would be her sit bones and hamstrings against the floor as she reached into a long Forward Fold.

Grounding put Amanda back into a close relationship with her body, which made it more difficult for her to abuse it with harmful behaviors like overeating, lack of movement, and aggressive self-talk. She slowly stopped punishing her body with neglect and negative talk, and her world began to change, too. She didn't end up dating the guy in the photo, but she found a boyfriend who loved her and helped her see her own beauty.

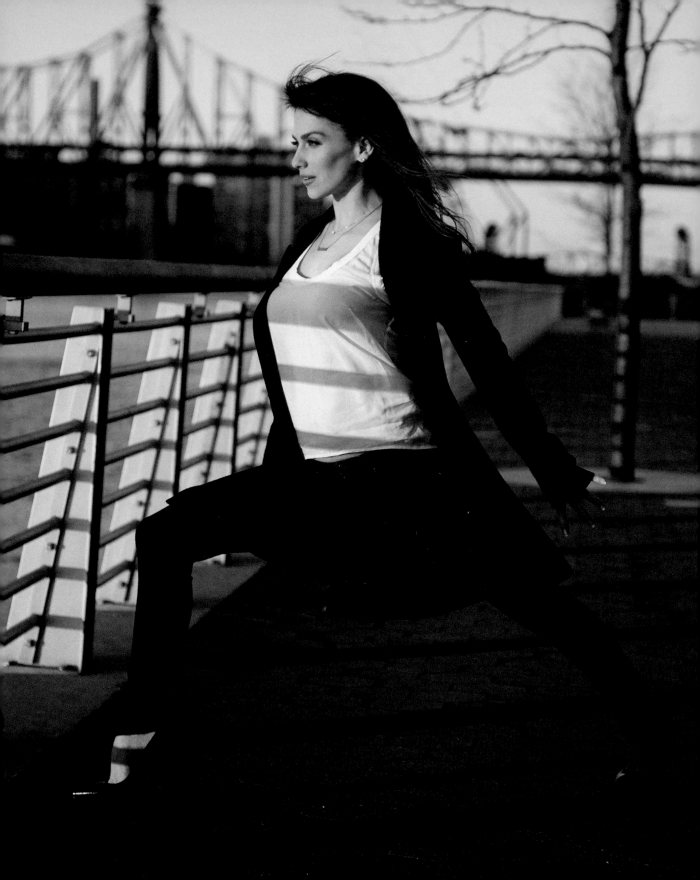

GRATITUDE FEEDS GROUNDING

Gratitude is a popular word these days. There are gratitude journals and gratitude calendars, books on gratitude, even gratitude apps. That's all fine and good, but you certainly don't have to purchase something to experience gratitude. When Living Clearly, it doesn't matter where or how you get your gratitude just as long as you get it. When you decide to turn on gratitude, you are instantly clicked out of your mind's winding list of what's not working in your life and into what's great about being you. This process brings you into the reality of your situation and plants you firmly in the seat of what's really happening.

The mind often skews negative. If you shined a spotlight on your inner dialogue at any time of the day, you might be shocked at how much time you spend complaining. Try it: For 1 whole day, note every time you catch yourself complaining. The complaints may be as insignificant as *This train is too crowded, this room is too hot, I feel tired or hungry or cranky*. Or more weighty—*Nobody loves me, I hate my job, the town I live in is uninspiring, I'll never succeed*. Even if you consider yourself a happy person and believe that your life is generally good, there's a strong chance that your complaining machine is still running on overdrive.

There's a famous proverb that says:

> *Be careful of your thoughts, for your thoughts become your words. Be careful of your words, for your words become your actions. Be careful of your actions, for your actions become your habits. Be careful of your habits, for your habits become your character. Be careful of your character, for your character becomes your destiny.*

If you swap complaints for positive observations, your world suddenly seems more enjoyable. It's more fun to be you. In the beginning, it may seem forced or awkward, but when it feels like everything is going wrong, I try to step back (perspective) and imagine how much worse it could be. This usually makes me stop and give it a chance. Complaining is really nothing more than a bad habit; by simply bringing awareness to it, you will slow the complaining and kick-start the changes that you want to see in your life. I halt and hit the reset button.

GRATITUDE EXERCISE

It's said that it takes 40 days for something to become a habit. Gratitude is a habit that is good for you and your life, so can you commit to 40 days of thankfulness? It's simple: For 40 consecutive days, jot down 10 things you're grateful for. No gratitude is too big or too small. You can go as micro as *There was no line at Starbucks when I rolled in for my morning coffee* or *It was nice and sunny today.* Or you can take note of bigger-picture items: *I'm healthy, I get to do work I love, I have amazing friends.*

Much like perspective and breathing, grounding is a Living Clearly tool that is there for you at the ready, whenever you need it. And the more you turn to it, cultivating a robust relationship with the felt experience of being in your body on the earth, the easier it will be for you to turn to it quickly and spontaneously. Practice it regularly, and turning on the principle will be second nature. It will be what you do when you need to come back to yourself.

Once you have become familiar with the sense of grounding, you can move into the next principle, balance. Finding a steady center point is impossible without first establishing a firm foundation to stand on.

Relevé

Relevé is a stealthy, effective method of grounding in any moment. You can do the exercise while standing anywhere. It's best practiced barefoot. Whenever you find yourself in a situation where you don't feel grounded, Relevé brings your attention to your feet on the ground, that unending source of security and foundation, remembering that you must press down in order to go up, rising up requests grounding. See detailed directions for Relevé in the Yoga for Grounding sequence on page 90.

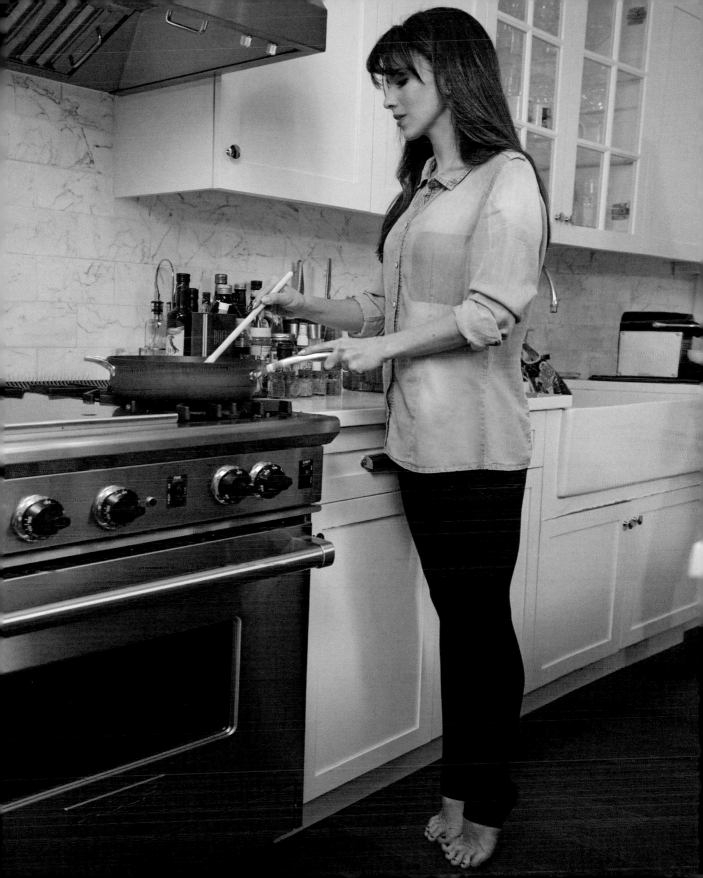

YOGA FOR GROUNDING

Every yoga pose provides an opportunity to experience grounding. Whether you're in Warrior 1 or Savasana, some part of your body is always in contact with the floor—or with another part of your body. We are beings who take comfort and find strength in stability and the sense of being supported. It is in this connection that the magic of grounding occurs. As you move through this sequence, pay special attention to the sensation of your feet or hands pressing into the floor or of your hands pressing into each other. The exchange of energy from surface to surface is what brings us into the present moment, and from there, you will be able to tap into increased vitality and stability. *Approximately 10 minutes.*

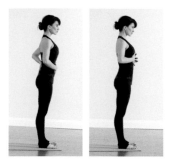 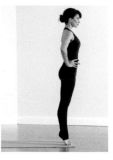 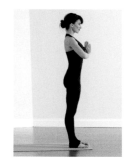

① Stand at the front of your mat in **TADASANA**. Take one hand to your belly and one to the base of your back. Draw your navel in toward your spine, activating your center. Place your hands onto your rib cage. Transition your hands to your hips and feel that you're pressing all of your body weight downward into your feet. Relax your shoulders down your back, focusing on your posture and on releasing your weight into the floor.

② Bring your hands to prayer position at your heart, and start to shift your body weight forward, coming onto the balls of your feet, pressing so firmly that your

heels start to peel off the floor into **RELEVÉ**. Always remember: Press down in order to go up, always moving up from the ground, which is a place of constant stability. You may feel unstable here. Your ankles may start to wobble, your legs may shake, and you might even fall over. This is all part of the practice. Keep feeling the balls of your feet grounding into the floor, and little by little, stability will come. When you're ready, release your heels to the floor, and then take two more rounds of **RELEVÉ**, inhaling the heels up and exhaling them down.

③ Bring your hands into a prayer at your heart center in **MOUNTAIN POSE**, and find your *ujjayi* breath.

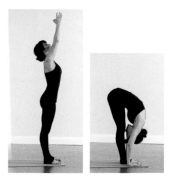

④ Inhale reach your hands above your head. Exhale **FORWARD FOLD**.

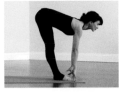

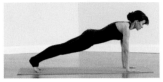

5 Inhale **HALF LIFT**. Exhale step your right foot back then your left foot into **PLANK POSE**.

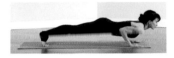

6 Inhale looking forward. Exhale **CHATURANGA**.

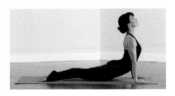

7 Inhale **UPWARD FACING DOG**, pressing into your hands.

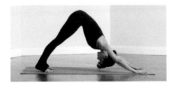

8 Exhale **DOWNWARD FACING DOG**, pushing the floor away, lifting your hips up, and bringing your heels low. Hold for five rounds of breath, grounding down through your hands and feet.

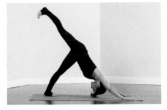

9 Press into your left foot to inhale your right leg up into **DOWNWARD FACING DOG SPLIT**.

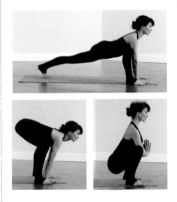

10 Exhale step your right foot to the outside of the right hand. Inhale step your left foot forward to the outside of the left hand. Exhale **SQUAT** down with your hands in a prayer at heart center. (If this is difficult for you, you can sit on a block or a very low chair. You can also roll up a blanket and place it under your heels.) Press your hands very firmly in toward one another to widen your elbows and deepen the hip stretch. Pull your belly button in while lengthening your spine. Always be aware of pressing into your feet to keep your core and spine long and strong.

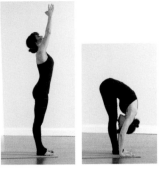

11 Ground and press into your feet as you straighten your legs, inhaling back up into **MOUNTAIN POSE**.

12 Exhale **FORWARD BEND**.

13 Inhale Half Lift. Exhale step your left foot back and then your right foot into **PLANK POSE**.

14 Inhale, look forward, exhale **CHATURANGA**.

15 Inhale **UPWARD DOG**. Exhale **DOWNWARD FACING DOG**. Take five rounds of breath. As you inhale, press your weight down through your hands, and as you exhale, ground down through your feet, pulling energy up from the floor.

Repeat on your left side, ending in Downward Facing Dog.

(continued)

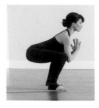

❶ Inhale your left leg up. Exhale step it to the outside of your left hand. Inhale step your right foot to the outside of your right hand. Exhale **HIGH SQUAT**. (This pose sits higher than a traditional squat.) Your pelvis and quads should be in alignment with your knees; you are making a 90-degree angle with the bend in your legs, and your pelvis should be more or less parallel with your mat. Your quads are in alignment with your knees. The core should be quite activated as your thighs fire up. Take three rounds of breath, relaxing your shoulders and pressing firmly into your feet to maintain the pose.

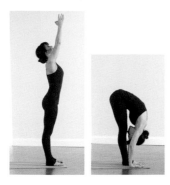

❷ Press into your feet as you inhale back up into **MOUNTAIN POSE**. Exhale. Fold over your legs.

❸ Inhale. Look forward into **HALF LIFT**. Exhale. **CHATURANGA**.

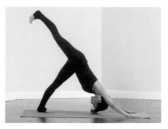

❹ Inhale **UPWARD DOG**. Exhale **DOWNWARD FACING DOG**. Inhale your right leg up into **DOWNWARD FACING DOG SPLIT**.

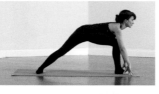

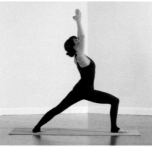

❺ Exhale step your right foot in between your hands, spiraling your back foot down at a 45-degree angle. Inhale **WARRIOR 1**.

❻ Exhale expand into **WARRIOR 2**, relaxing your shoulders down your back, open your hips up to feel your weight releasing downward into the floor.

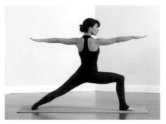

Make sure the front knee is over the ankle. Reach long through the arms, maximizing the distance between the right and left hands. Hold for five breaths.

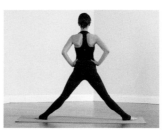

❼ Inhale straighten your front leg. Exhale turn your right toes in a little and your left toes out a little so that you are making a small, turned-out V shape (don't turn out too much; this is not ballet). Inhale take your hands to your waist. Exhale lower into **GODDESS POSE**, with your legs wider than your mat, feet pointing slightly out.

❽ Inhale and tip your body weight forward. Slide your hands from your hips down your inner thighs so they rest just before your knees. Exhale press your left hand— this is a grounding action— into your left thigh and twist toward the right in **WIDE GODDESS TWIST**.

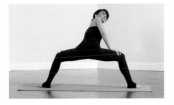

With every inhale and exhale, deepen into the twist, opening up through your hips and stretching up through your spine. Feel your feet strong on the ground. Take five rounds of breath.

9 Inhale, come to center, straightening your legs, and exhale **WARRIOR 2** on the right side,

10 Inhale bring your hands to the floor, framing your front foot. Exhale **CHATURANGA**. As you lower down, feel yourself resisting the floor, grounding with your hands and feet.

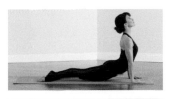

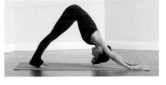

11 Inhale **UPWARD DOG**. Exhale **DOWNWARD FACING DOG**.

Repeat on your left side.

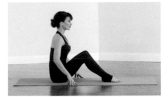

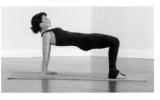

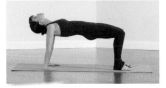

1 Sit on your butt, with your knees bent and hip-distance apart and your feet on the floor. Bring your hands (fingertips facing forward) on your mat behind you. Inhale **TABLE TOP**, pressing into your feet and hands. (This pose is great for toning your legs and butt.) Keep your chin tucked, looking at your knees. If you can raise your pelvis high enough so that you lose sight of your knees, you can release your chin and head back, looking upward. As you practice grounding, always be aware of where your body is touching the floor. Look toward your knees. Take five rounds of breath.

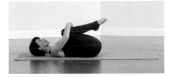

2 Lie on your back and draw your knees into your chest, coming into **APANASANA**. Wrap your arms around your legs (the more you draw your knees into your chest, the more you release your lower back). Take five rounds of breath.

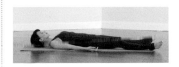

3 Come into **SAVASANA**. Release completely. The floor will catch you. Imagine gravity cloaking you like a blanket, assisting you in your release. Scan your body to see where you are still holding any tension. Bring your attention to which points of your body are in contact with the floor. Notice how with each inhale and exhale, those points deepen and increase in number. Inhale into the muscles that are still holding. Exhale the tension out. Remember that we crave stability and grounding for our own well-being. You can conjure up so much strength and relieve tremendous stress here simply by releasing your body weight down. Take 3 to 5 minutes.

Your hand opens and closes, opens and closes. If it were always a fist or always stretched open, you would be paralyzed. Your deepest presence is in every small contracting and expanding, the two as beautifully balanced and coordinated as birds' wings.

—RUMI

Chapter Seven

THE FOURTH PRINCIPLE

BALANCE

THERE WILL BE PERIODS OF YOUR LIFE WHEN THE SCALE TIPS. SOMETHING has pulled you too far to one side—excessive exercise, excessive eating, excessive lack of rest, excessive laziness—and has caused you to lose your footing, allowing an extreme state to take over. We've all been there. This slipping away from equilibrium is a natural part of being human. We are fluid creatures, ever changing and transforming, and swinging toward excess is part of our ways. When we fall out of balance, we lose the ability to make good decisions; we become fractured, burdened, and unclear. This is why our society is *obsessed* with balance! From magazine headlines pushing us to strike a work life balance to nutritionists imploring us to eat a balanced diet, we're clearly all yearning for greater equilibrium.

After experiencing the painful results of living a life out of balance, I keep my antennae especially attuned to my own state of equilibrium. Before I met Alec and became a mother, my weak spot was overactivity. I would just do too much, too hard, too many days of the week (well, all of them, really). I put my body through the ringer. I was immersed in yoga—teaching it, practicing it, and running a yoga studio—but that wasn't enough. I was still running most days, dancing, and maintaining a full social life. I had little perspective; it felt like the end of the world if I missed a yoga class, resting seemed like a waste of time, and self-care was silly and indulgent. And this incessant action and unbalanced lifestyle landed me in a wheelchair.

Today, demands come at me from caring for my children, supporting my husband's career, cultivating my own creative projects, taking care of my body, and nurturing my marriage. Some days it feels like I'm hitting balls from one of those automatic tennis ball machines: lob, whack, lob, whack. Sometimes I miss, for sure, putting too much time into one thing, hyperfocusing on one part of my life and neglecting another. Too much work and not enough rest, and I get sick. Too much time with the kids and not enough with Alec, and we argue. Too much time working and not enough time exercising, and I get out of sorts. This hard-won understanding serves me well because my life is more full

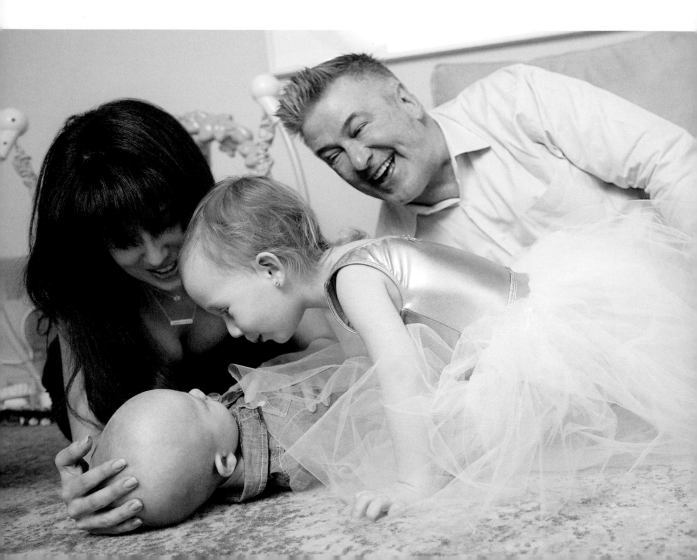

now than I could have ever imagined. But there's always another ball right behind the one I just swung at and missed, another chance to practice balance and the rest of the Living Clearly Principles.

Balance is fundamental yet so easy to lose. Lean just a bit too much in one direction and, whoosh, you've lost your footing, and well-being and ease suddenly vanish. I see it all the time in my clients' lives and in my own life. Drink one too many glasses of wine and you're hungover the next day; say something hurtful during an argument with a loved one and you're filled with regret. Balance is elusive, slipping through your fingers before you realize it. This is normal and expected. Swinging in and out of the center point is actually part of the process of balancing.

Like the micro shifts you make in Tree Pose or any other balancing posture in yoga, living a life in balance requires an ongoing series of small and subtle adjustments to help you maintain equilibrium.

Balance also requires thoughtful and consistent attention to your own state of well-being; you have to know what you need before you can see what's missing. You must first recognize that you've lost your center, and this can feel scary and overwhelming or make you cranky and stressed. Practicing the first three principles is a simple method of inquiry, a surefire way of getting to know yourself. Gaining perspective allows you to see the bigger picture of your life, breathing whisks you into the present moment so you can see what's really happening, and grounding welcomes you deeply into the home of your body, where you can feel safe and rooted in yourself.

> You have to know what you need before you can see what's missing.

I find that my relationship with Alec gives me the greatest opportunity to practice balance. Like any married couple, we sometimes bicker and argue—often over silly things. And because we both have strong personalities, our fights have the potential to escalate quickly; before we know it, we're both agitated and then angry and resentful. These days, though, we rarely move into hurtful arguments. As we continually integrate each principle into our lives, we find that the work is contagious. The more we actively tune in to our reactivity, the harder it is for one of us to get into a conflict. When I feel things start to get stressful between us, when I see that one or both of us is triggered and tempers are starting to flare, I bring my attention specifically to balance; I attempt to do this in any conflict situation I encounter.

(continued on page 100)

Dancer's Pose

When I talk about balance, Dancer's Pose is always one of the first poses that I mention. This pose is the ultimate study in balance; there you are on one foot with the other foot pressed into your hand, extending behind your body. This is an excellent pose to improve your falling skills. Yes, you can be good at falling! Every yogi has landed in an awkward pile on the floor in one pose or another over the course of her practice. Falling is humbling, sure, and embarrassing (it shouldn't be), but it's one of the best and least subtle metaphors for getting through life. A lot of people fall over in Dancer's Pose, especially if you are doing it in stilettos on a windy spring day on the top of a huge building. (You know how many times I fell trying to get this picture?). Mostly because they're thinking about the shape of it instead of the specific recipe of movements required to make it a reality. It's too cerebral; there's no way I can maintain this position. Then, boom, fall, crash, I'm on the floor. In life, when you push yourself too hard, try to take on too many tasks, or overthink a project, something will slip through the cracks and you are bound to fumble. The brain is the absolute worst place to be in a balancing pose. The more you think, the harder it will be.

I use a game of tug-of-war as a metaphor for the tautness that's essential in Dancer's Pose. To know where your center is, you've got to have an understanding of equally opposing forces. I have students place their foot in their hand and, before leaning forward, kick back, pressing their foot firmly into their hand and feeling that force. They should feel an intense stretch through the front of the working shoulder and potentially through the bent leg's psoas. Only then can they lean forward, just an inch at a time. Kick a little into the hand, lean a little forward, kick a little more, and lean a little more. It is a balanced, 50/50 action. The entire process is supported by a bright and active core, because feeling your center over your standing foot keeps you steady and strong. When it's time to come out of the pose, simply move yourself in the opposite direction, bringing your leg forward to propel your torso back up to a standing position. Keep pressing your foot into your hand while bringing your knees together, feeling the taut tension between your leg and hand, just like a game of tug-of-war where both ends of the rope are being pulled equally. When students do it this way, they rarely fall—though falling is always okay.

DANCER'S POSE

Stand on your right foot and bring your left elbow to your hip. Reach back and grab onto the inside of your left foot with your thumb facing toward your big toe. Slowly kick your foot into your hand and as your body tilts forward an inch or two, continue to push your foot into your hand to counter the forward movement. Little by little, tilt your body forward even more while simultaneously kicking back (these are equally opposing movements). Note the grounding occurring between your hand and your back foot and between your right foot and the floor. Activate your core as you gently seek balance.

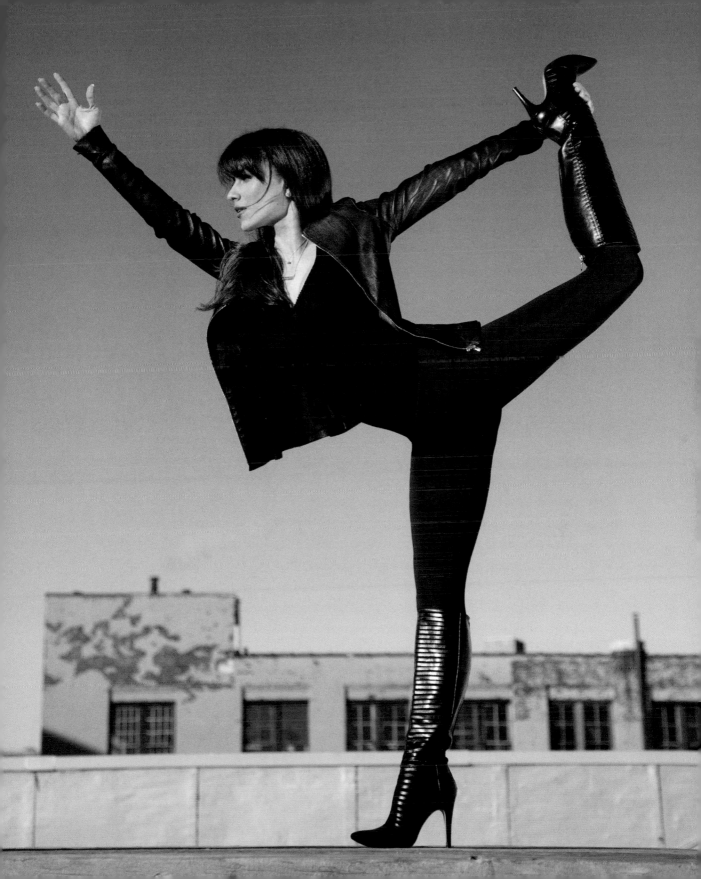

I picture arguments like being on a seesaw. Each person is trying to force his/her side of it and win, pushing violently with his/her feet to force the other person to come crashing into the earth! Instead of doing that, I try to visualize myself standing at the middle point of the seesaw between the two sides—between my desire to be right and win and the other person's urge to dominate the argument. If I can remain steady in the middle, which requires an activation of my core and subtle adjustments to stay firmly rooted, both sides get to hover at equal height, and now we can try to see eye-to-eye. Standing in the middle of the seesaw doesn't mean that I am subverting my own needs, not standing by my beliefs, or allowing the other person to walk all over me. The middle isn't caving in; in fact, striking balance like that is actually deeply empowering.

If I remained stuck in my own experience, forcing my side of the seesaw to the ground, I would be overcome with challenging emotions. I would be lost in a sea of resentment and contempt, and the things I really care about would be fuzzy and out of focus. When arguing with Alec, I could forget that we love each other very much, that we are committed to each other's happiness, and that he is permitted to have feelings and opinions that differ from mine. By remaining balanced, at the center of the seesaw, I stay true to myself, honoring my own needs while respecting and honoring his position, as well.

Resisting the magnetic pull to be right takes strength and a fiery activation of your center. But it gets easier with practice. Soon, dropping the need to be right will be uplifting and empowering. Plus, if you really love and care for someone, you want them to feel good and validated too, right? There is a notable shift that happens when I strike a balance during an argument (this is the contagious part!). By simply initiating a move toward the middle, by relinquishing the need to be right, the temperature begins to cool and I see Alec begin to relax, move out of his own defensive posture, and open toward me again. He can see that I'm not trying to win, that it's actually not about winning or losing, that it's about finding a new way to relate to each other and making everyone happy.

HARNESSING CORE POWER

When we tap into our core, we connect with our emotional strength as well as our physical strength. People come to the mat with everything they have experienced so far—their victories, traumas, all of it. Often I can sense what they are carrying by the way they activate, or don't activate, their core on the mat. Like Julia, a former student of mine. She

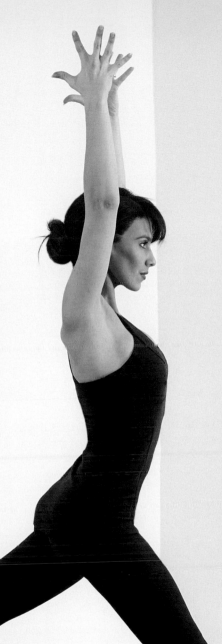

Moving High Lunge

Moving High Lunge (see page 107 in the Yoga for Balance sequence for more instructions on this pose) is a study in balance. There's no way you can be in it, clicked into proper alignment, and not feel powerful and alive. This posture requires strong effort from the quads, but it is far from all legs. To really make this pose come alive, you must energize your core. It is the activation of your center that allows you to shine brightly in all directions. Your arms are reaching up toward the sky, your front foot and back heel are rooting toward the earth, your tailbone sinks down, and your head is tall and proud. As you bend and release your front knee in this moving posture, your legs are working, but it is the energy of your core that supports the process.

As you bring your attention to your core in the balancing poses in this chapter, begin to distinguish the softness of your stomach from the firmness of the muscles that surround it. It's a brilliant contrast. The softness represents your emotional state; it is humility and compassion (I am relaxed, present, and grateful). The strength is the way you bring those qualities to the world (I am confident, clear, and focused). While in Moving High Lunge, feel the crown of your head tall and proud while your tailbone and spine move in separate directions like a bungee cord. Bring your attention to the energy of your center. Feel yourself making subtle adjustments, maybe wobbling a bit from side to side, and then finding the middle point again. Finally, bring your attention to your feet. They should be soft and wide. Feel all four corners of each foot rooting firmly down into the mat. Don't grip your toes; spread them out, creating a soft, stable surface to balance on.

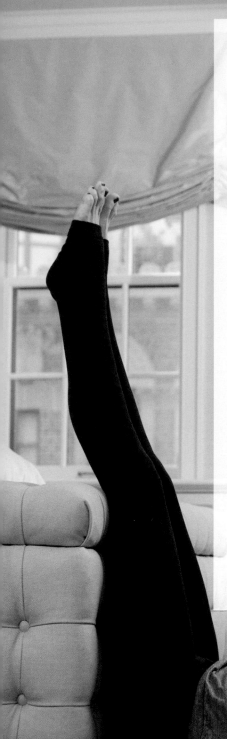

Feet Up the Wall

We balance on our feet all day—walking, running, hopping, skipping—but our true sense of balance comes from the middle point of the body, halfway between the head and the toes. This powerhouse of energy and centeredness is our core. While our society is obsessed with a flat stomach, the image is a superficial one of rock-hard washboard abs, not one of powerful centered energy. Gymnastics, dance, and yoga are wildly different practices, but when I got to know each intimately, I discovered that they all rely on a strong and powerful core. When the core is strong and activated, you can move the body with more control and grace. Your movements are infused with intention, focused and on target; it's a lot harder to fall on your face when your core is activated and alive.

A truly energized core taps into several muscle groups, all equally important. There is the rectus abdominis, the most external of the core muscles and the source of all that ab attention (you feel these muscles when you do any kind of crunching exercise). Then there are the obliques, which run diagonal along the flank of the body, attaching to the midline beneath the rectus abdominis, and they are key players in stabilizing the torso in lateral standing poses. There's also the transverse abdominis, a band of muscle that holds the contents of the abdomen in place; the adductors, a group of muscles that connect the thighbone to the pelvis; quadratus lumborum, a deeper muscle that connects the upper and lower bodies and is a bit harder to feel but plays a key role in standing poses; and finally, psoas major, which is a hip flexor that sits across the pelvis in front of the pubic bone and attaches from the lumbar spine to the inner thighbone. While lying on the floor, scoot your butt aside a wall, chair, or ottoman, with the legs pointing up. Or you can even bend and rest the legs on the chair or ottoman.

was a young woman in her twenties who would hire me to teach semi-private classes a couple times a week with her girlfriends. They were fun and enthusiastic, really interested in technique and mastery of new poses. Julia moved through my classes easily but struggled with inversions, any pose that required her to lift her legs above her head, even in a gentle pose like Feet Up the Wall. Whenever I tried to guide her into the pose, she would start hyperventilating, kick her legs as though she was being attacked, and curl up on her side, looking terrified. I told her that she didn't have to do the pose if it brought up such a strong reaction, but she was determined and insisted on practicing it regularly. She wasn't fearful in other postures, and it seemed clear to me that her block was emotional. I suggested that we work together one-on-one, and she agreed.

When we met, I started her off with a small flow sequence, connecting her body, breath, and movement. Then we sat together, and I asked her if she knew why she struggled so much with inversions. We had developed trust over the past year, and she burst into tears as she told me that she had been raped several years ago and had never told anyone. It was someone she knew, a date gone very wrong. There was too much alcohol, too much force, and not enough listening when she told him to stop. As she was sobbing, I asked her to lie down and close her eyes. I had her place one hand on her belly and the other on her chest. She gripped the hand on her belly, pulling at the skin and writhing in emotional pain. She had lost the ability to connect to her center, which made her unable to balance or feel comfortable when her feet weren't on the ground.

Through our work together, she began to slowly reconnect to her core. I would ask her to focus on bringing her naval toward her spine, which is one way to activate the center. I was sure to keep this part light and fun, focusing more on the physical aspects of things, getting her to sweat and really feel her body. But I knew that this deep level of core-centered practice would also help her find her way back to a solid sense of herself. Being violated so invasively had fractured her confidence, and building core strength was rebuilding this fundamental aspect of her being. This process is what the poet E. E. Cummings would call the moment you feel you are nobody but yourself.

Restorative poses (such as child's pose, supta baddha konasana/reclining goddess, or savasana) were a big part of our practice, and during our time together, I also suggested that she seek counseling for victims of rape, which she did. While she was in these gentle poses, we would talk about what happened to her, and I would bring her attention to how her body was responding to her words. I would guide her slowly through the story, continually bringing her physical and mental focus back to her hand on her heart and her hand on her belly. After several weeks, she was no longer gripping, there was no more tearing at her flesh. With her hand on her center, she learned to feel her body again, to remember who she was, and to tap into her worthiness to soften her center, her being, her feeling of balance.

Today, Julia is still one of my star group students. Now, she can easily bring her feet up the wall and even do a shoulder stand on her own at the end of class. She has continued with rape counseling and now volunteers with rape victims, as well. She is a special soul who worked to find her core, and from there, chose life, and herself.

As you'll see when practicing Tree Pose, balancing poses require alignment, core strength, and attention. Drop any one of them and you'll fall out of the position. If you are tipped too far to one side (out of alignment), you won't be able to hold the pose. If you don't activate your core, you will crumble into yourself, and if your attention wanders—you start thinking about what you're going to have for dinner or what the person is doing next to you—your pose doesn't stand a chance. *Drishti,* or focused gaze, is an essential component of all balancing yoga poses in that it channels your attention. When your eyes are calm, your mind will be calm, too. After you move into the balancing pose, find a point in front of you that you can softly rest your gaze on. This point becomes your anchor, but it's not necessary to grip onto it desperately. Just as you're continually adjusting and readjusting your pose, finding your center and then losing it and then coming back again, you will drop your *drishti* and then come back to it.

> Balancing poses require alignment, core strength, and attention. Drop any one of them and you'll fall out of the position.

When I start to feel pulled off center by opposing forces—which I do, often—I practice balancing poses. I hone in on my core, using the action of my body as a roadway back to my center. Consistently practicing tapping into your core helps you get back to your center in any situation. Regardless of how full your plate may be, don't let go of your core; it is your home base, your shelter from any storm.

Now, empowered with perspective, breathing, grounding, and balance, you are prepared to move into the final Living Clearly principle, the place of ultimate release and surrender, letting go.

Steady Like a Tree

Many yoga poses take their inspiration from nature, turning to the shapes of plants and animals. Tree Pose is one of my favorites to teach because it has a quick learning curve and brings deep satisfaction and strength to those who can master it. Trees are incredible teachers. They can be old and majestic—think of some of the redwoods of California—or quite young and delicate, like a little sapling planted in a city park. Either way, they are in a continuous state of balance, reaching up to the sky with their trunks and branches and deep into the earth with their complex root systems. And like us, trees must brave the changing elements of their environment, adapting to windy, stormy, or cold climates and transforming with the seasons.

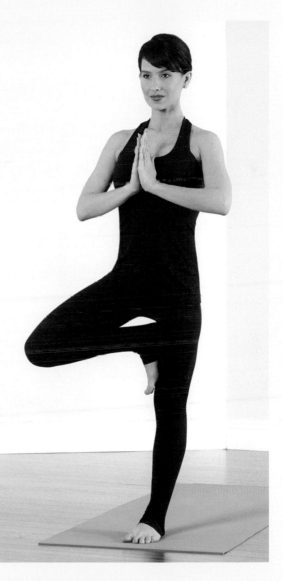

In yoga, Tree is also an adaptable pose. You can adjust it to fit your mood and ability, keeping it soft and simple with your hands on your waist and one foot pressed low on your calf or more energized and dynamic with one foot pressed into the top of your inner thigh, your arms reaching tall and wide, and your chin poised up. Whatever variation you choose, Tree requires an activation of your core. If you move into the pose using only muscular effort from your legs or arms, you will fall over.

YOGA FOR BALANCE

Yoga gives us so many opportunities to experiment with balance. As you move through the various balancing postures in this sequence—all different, but each requiring a fired-up core and a playful spirit—give yourself room to feel your edges, to get shaky and wobbly, to fall down and get back up again. Yoga is not a perfect practice. It is a safe place to see how gravity works and to notice where you strike balance easily and where it is more challenging to stay steady. Allow yourself to ask, *How is my body balanced over and in between the points that are touching the floor? Approximately 10 minutes*

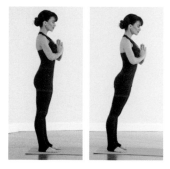

❶ Stand at the back of your mat in **MOUNTAIN POSE**, with your hands at your heart in prayer. Place your feet hip-distance apart. Close your eyes and shift your weight slightly forward and slightly back, to the left and to the right. Really feel where the weight is distributed over and between your feet. We rely greatly on our eyes for balance, but releasing sight is a valuable lesson as balance is primarily about feeling. The eyes can assist, but if you don't tap into the feeling in your body, you won't be able to balance. Play around with shifting your weight for 1 to 2 minutes.

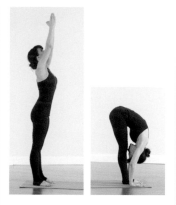

❷ Open your eyes, inhale, reach your prayer hands up toward the ceiling. As you exhale, **FORWARD FOLD**.

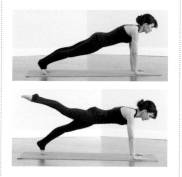

❸ Inhale, walk your hands forward into **PLANK POSE**, and lift your right leg up. Hold for five rounds of breath. Notice how lifting

your leg shifts the weight distribution over your hands and your feet as it changes your balance. You have to engage your core to maintain the pose. *(Option: Place your left knee on your mat.)*

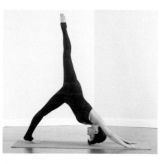

❹ Inhale, press through your hands, and move straight back into **DOWNWARD FACING DOG SPLIT** with your right leg up.

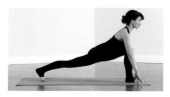

❺ Exhale step your foot through into **LOW LUNGE**. Inhale High Lunge and straighten your front knee.

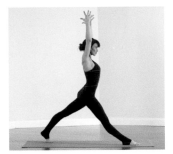

Exhale bend it back to a 90-degree angle. Inhale straighten, exhale bend. This is **MOVING HIGH LUNGE**. Straighten and bend your knee for five rounds of breath.

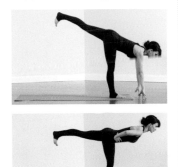

6 Inhale your hands to the floor. Exhale step onto your front foot, raising up your back leg. Come onto your fingertips, and then slowly bring your hands to your hips in **WARRIOR 3** (for extra support, your hands may be on the floor, blocks, or a piece of furniture). Try to parallel your chest to the floor, feeling your back leg rotate in so your toes are flexed and pointing down toward the floor. Your back heel and your chest should be in one straight line, creating a T with your body.

(It's totally okay to wobble here. If you don't fall, you won't get any better!) Hold the pose for five rounds of breath.

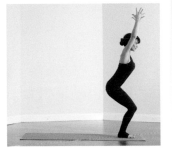

7 Inhale **CHAIR POSE**, bringing your left leg in to meet your right. Exhale soften your shoulders down your back. Notice the relief of having two feet on the floor, but also note the intensity of this pose. Hold the pose for five rounds of breath.

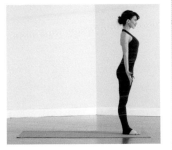

8 Inhale **MOUNTAIN POSE**. Exhale release your hands by your sides in **SAMASTHITI**.

9 Step onto your left foot, preparing for **TREE POSE**. Bend your right knee into your chest, butterfly your knee open, and press the sole of your foot either above or below your knee. You can

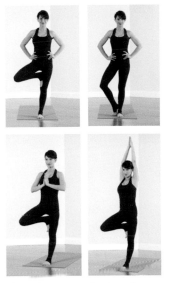

also place your foot on the floor by your ankle. Bring your hands to your heart in a prayer or on your hips. *(Option: Reach your hands up to the ceiling, arms extended.)* Take three rounds of breath.

10 Inhale your knee to point forward. Exhale your foot down on the ground, and bring your arms by your sides in **SAMASTHITI**. Inhale reach your arms up.

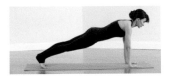

11 Exhale **FORWARD BEND**. Inhale **HALF LIFT**. Exhale step back into **PLANK POSE**.

Repeat on your left side. After Tree Pose on your left side, finish in Mountain Pose.

I want to know if you can be alone with yourself and if you truly like the company you keep in the empty moments.

—ORIAH, *THE INVITATION*

Chapter Eight

THE FIFTH PRINCIPLE
LETTING GO

IT'S AN ALMOST ICONIC IMAGE THESE DAYS: A ROOMFUL OF YOGIS LYING flat on their backs, arms and legs spread wide, eyes closed, sinking into their final relaxation after a vigorous class of Downward Facing Dogs and Warrior 1s. With absolutely no muscular effort involved, Corpse Pose is the cherry on top of your yoga workout, the reward for all that exertion and sweating. So how come so few people can actually do the pose correctly? Sure, all those supine yogis *look* relaxed, but if you could peek into the mind inside any one of those bodies "resting" on the floor, you'd discover a landscape that's as busy and bustling as Times Square.

Savasana is said to be the hardest yoga pose of the bunch, and with good reason. One of the most common yoga-related misunderstandings that people approach me with is that they think there is a prerequisite to turn their minds completely off during practice. Now, this is something that many yoga instructors will actually teach—however, in my approach, we respect and accept that the mind absolutely loves to be busy. It always made me feel uncomfortable to tell people to clear their minds and just let the body take over because it goes completely against the mind's constitution. The mind absolutely loves to be busy. Ask it to solve a problem like getting the fritzy Wi-Fi to work, untangling a stubborn knot, or figuring out how to move you through a series of complex yoga poses and it happily reports for duty, trying to conceptualize how to get your right foot in one place while your left foot makes its way all the way over there. When we approach a restorative pose like Savasana, the mind often rebels and feels uncomfortable with the seemingly motionless state the body has found its way into. A fidgety fear sets in, as many teachers tell their students to clear their minds completely. In my philosophy, we acknowledge the mind's chatty character yet try to redirect its busy, all-over-the-place, bad stressed-out habits by giving it a job to do during Savasana. We encourage the mind to focus on the sensations of release in the body. This is something that most of us don't do enough. We rarely focus on actually relaxing, unwinding our stressed-out muscles, and find a way into a healthier state. Give the mind a problem to solve and it is happy; tell the mind to go away, and it will rebel. By bringing the body into a restorative, releasing posture, and teaching the mind to assist in its release, we are able to achieve calming both the body and the mind at the same time. After all, the whole point of yoga is connecting the mind and the body. It is surprising how much we are actually still clenching when we think we have released into a calming pose. A misunderstanding that a lot of people have is assuming that once the body is in the position, we have accomplished our goal. But Savasana isn't about creating the assumed position of release, it is about actually attaining letting go. It's a process. When I assume this posture, I scan the body: What am I still holding on to? Can I relax my shoulders a bit more? Can I release my jaw? How about my brow? Little by little the body lets go and the mind gets wrapped up in the difficult job of unwinding tension. Both are completely consumed by the task at hand. And it is a calming task. One of finding complete peace and unity from within.

So let the mind be busy, but direct it toward a path of health and happiness. Let both it and the body be the recipients of the wonderful gifts of de-stressing. No boredom suffered in the process!

Letting go is the culmination of the Five Living Cleary Principles, and Savasana is the

> *Stillness is our most intense mode of action. It is in our moments of deep quiet that is born every idea, emotion, and drive which we eventually honor with the name of action. We reach highest in meditation, and farthest in prayer. In stillness every human being is great.*
>
> **—LEONARD BERNSTEIN**

ultimate physical representation of the act of letting go. The yoga poses and exercises in the first four principle chapters are designed to prepare you for this final step on the path to Living Clearly by encouraging your mind to get out of the driver's seat and giving your body permission to take the lead. By experiencing each principle physically, you are able to imprint its essence into your being. Perhaps you experienced this while stretching tall into Tree Pose, wobbling, regaining equilibrium, maybe falling, getting up again, until you were finally able to sense that precious moment when you struck balance, and then from there, hopefully, you were able to carry that feeling into your everyday life. The same goes for Corpse Pose, which uses the body to show the mind what it feels like to fully release. But as you'll likely discover while practicing Savasana and the other letting-go poses in this chapter, truly letting go is a lot harder than it looks.

In countless yoga classes, I've witnessed thousands of people fidget and fumble and force their way around and eventually into final relaxation. Having been one of those buzzing, busy urbanites myself, I get it. After 75 minutes of sweating and stretching, moving your muscles, ligaments, and bones through space into new and different positions, it can be really challenging to come to a hard stop. And after a day—or a week or a lifetime—of plotting, strategizing, worrying, or obsessing, slowing down can seem all but impossible.

But why? I vividly remember my own experiences as a newbie yogi. After a lifetime in the hyperstimulating worlds of dance and gymnastics, and after making it through the foreign terrain of a Sanskrit-laden yoga class, the final relaxation at the end was anything but relaxing. My body would be splayed out flat on the mat, but my mind would still be whizzing from all it was asked to consider during class. I would to-do list my way through every minute of Savasana. I'd make my grocery list, review all I had to do that night and the next day, draft e-mails, script future conversations. It didn't matter how calming the music was or how sweetly the teacher walked us through releasing each part of the body; my mind would not let go, and so my body remained tense, too.

When I started working one-on-one with students, I recognized my early Savasana experiences in the fitful way they approached the pose. I let my students know that they could be open with me about what was happening for them when they attempted to get quiet in final relaxation and, in doing so, discovered some universal obstacles to letting go. Simply stated, really letting go is about being able to accept the messages you receive when you get quiet enough for your body and your heart to be heard. Often, when you strip away the noise and distractions and get really, really still, you can hear something

Savasana

Being a New York City yoga instructor has given me the opportunity to people watch extensively. Sometimes I would teach about 700 people a day! I've learned so much about how human beings function just by watching what happens in class, especially at the end of class. Many yoga students are resistant to Savasana, especially the fitness junkies. They've come to my class to sweat, flex, and tone, and just when things are really heating up, I ask them to lay it all down in Corpse Pose. Some people just can't stop moving, their fingers tapping to any music that's playing. Some keep their eyes open, checking out what's happening in the room, and some pass out cold. You don't have to do it one way. You can lie flat with your hands by your side, with your palms up. You can have one hand on your heart and one on your belly. You can skip lying down altogether and take a seated meditation if that's what feels right. I want you to choose the posture that will best help you release. All I ask as a teacher is that you give yourself a pose that will bring closure to your practice. For me, Savasana is the completion of everything. After stretching and sweating, these are the 5 minutes that bring it all together, where you get to let go and sink into the results of your effort.

that makes you uncomfortable, a feeling or sense of knowing that has been pushed into a dark corner. On the outside it may look as if you have an ideal life, with happy kids and a supportive, loving spouse, but if deep on the inside you know that your partner isn't right for you, there's a good chance that you won't be able to ignore that information when you get quiet in a letting-go pose. I believe that most of us avoid silence and stillness, whether in letting-go poses like Savasana or in meditation, because there is something inside of us that we don't want to face.

I see it all the time in my students in Manhattan. Many of them are externally successful, shining on the surface, but just below lurks a question that leads to a truth that is itching to be heard: *I'm showing up, going through the motions, but am I really happy?* The good news is that the simple act of becoming aware of a hurt place inside of you begins the process of resolution. If we are courageous enough to let our fears have a voice, they begin to move through us and heal. The longer you avoid, ignore, or deny what's true for you, the more the tender spot will grow inside you. Luckily, like all of the Living Clearly Principles, letting go gets easier with practice.

THE RSR PROCESS

The action of letting go is subtle. Think of letting go of a small rock that you're holding in your hand. You simply open your fingers and it releases to the ground. There is minimal muscular effort; you're not throwing it or clutching it. But when practiced regularly, letting go is an incredibly powerful way to take care of yourself. When we are experts at letting go, we become less fearful about giving up things that are not working or not necessary, clearing the way so that we engage in what really matters. This could be in a relationship with another person or in prioritizing all the things that need to be accomplished in our lives. When you are adept at letting go, you organically pick and choose your battles. Practicing letting go creates more ease in your life; there is less struggle, less forcing, less longing for something to be other than it is.

Whether you're on your mat or in real life, letting go is a simple three-step process, something I like to call the RSR Process: release, surrender, receive. You can practice RSR in the letting-go poses in this chapter and at any moment in life when you're feeling the need for a greater sense of ease, like when circumstances seem particularly charged or forced.

Release

Letting go is first and foremost about releasing the tension and stress of challenging situations. When in Savasana, you can practice release by dropping any "shoulds" that you've brought with you into the pose. *I should be able to relax. I should be better at Corpse Pose (it's Corpse Pose after all!). I should come to class more often. I should be doing something else.* Release them as you would sheets of paper into an open flame, allowing them to be quickly consumed and turned to ash. Visualize this as you sink deeper into Savasana. The key question here is, *What would this situation look like without the added stress or anxiety?* It's great to practice release when you feel yourself beginning to worry about somebody else. If your teenager doesn't come home on time, you can quickly get swept away in fearful thoughts, the swirling vortex of what-ifs. Or you can release the buzzing anxiety, shedding it like a snake sheds skin that no longer fits, so you can see and think clearly and take decisive action. Without tension and stress clouding your vision, you calmly find out the name and time of the movie your daughter attended and call her closest friends for a status report.

Surrender

Letting go can't happen unless you surrender deeply into your own reality. This requires a focus in two directions: on what is already good, beautiful, and working in your life *and* on the places where you can grow, stretch, or improve. Just as your center remained strong and soft simultaneously while working toward balance, you carry that duality with you into letting go. The Living Clearly journey of getting to know yourself has hopefully positioned you to be able to see what is excellent about yourself and your life (need a refresher? revisit the Gratitude Exercise on page 88) and to see what is holding you back (think: negative self-talk and unhealthy habits). As you surrender to what is real, you will be in an ideal position to see what is keeping you from moving forward. When in Savasana, surrender is the sweet experience of being held. As you sink into the floor, feel it holding you up firmly; it's a reliable and trustworthy foundation. You can stop all holding, gripping, grasping, or longing and just be, exactly as you are, and know that you won't fall. I find that this aspect of letting go is especially wonderful for mothers or those who are caretakers. Now it's our turn to be held.

Pigeon Pose

Pigeon Pose is a subtly powerful letting-go pose. It may look relaxing (and for those with open hips, it usually is), but it gets right into the hip flexors and rotators and can also release tension in the lower back. Pigeon is especially beneficial for people who sit a lot or drive a lot, as sedentary activities can wreak havoc on the hips, tightening them intensely. Active sports like cycling or running can also be hard on the hips, so sporty types also benefit from Pigeon. If you are seeking a more engaged pose but still want to experience letting go, Pigeon could be just what you need.

While you're in Pigeon, bring your attention to the fine balance between feeling challenged by the stretch and having it be just too hard. If the pose is too difficult, your body will naturally begin to resist what's happening and will create tension rather than a sense of letting go. With every inhale, ask yourself, *What am I activating in my body?* And with every exhale, ask yourself, *Can I let go a little more?*

See detailed instructions on moving into Pigeon Pose on page 126 in the Yoga for Letting Go sequence and for variations if this pose is too intense.

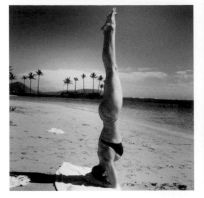
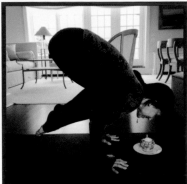
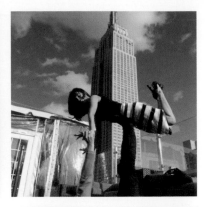
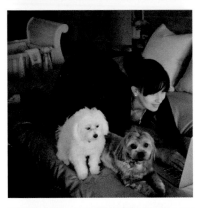
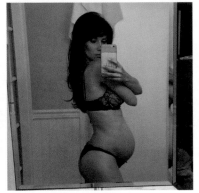
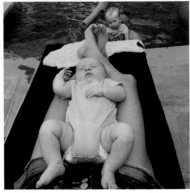
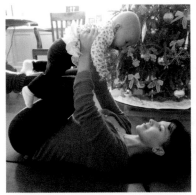
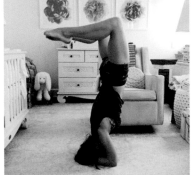
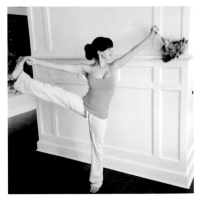
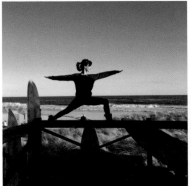
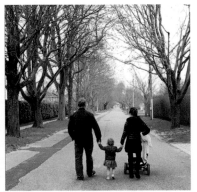
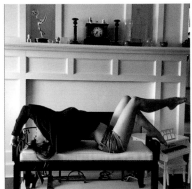

Receive

The final step of the letting-go process is receiving. When you truly let go, you are soft and open; there is nothing forced or rigid about your body or mind (just try to let something go with a tight belly or clenched jaw). And when you let go of the need to be right, you're quickly filled with compassion for another's experience. Let go of anger, and you're filled with understanding, kindness, or love. Let go of things looking one way, and you open yourself up to greater possibilities. In Savasana, you are set up to receive. On your back, arms and heart open, you are vulnerable and available to the world, there to take in what's bright, vibrant, and healthy while letting go of what's negative, dark, or not useful.

HOW I USE SOCIAL MEDIA TO PRACTICE LETTING GO

By choosing to expose myself on social media, I open myself up to the thoughts and opinions of many people that I will never meet in person, a position that is often quite vulnerable. I started my Instagram account with the hope that it would be a place of learning and community for women around the world who were interested in improving their health, strengthening their bodies, or just feeling more connected and less alone. I made a commitment to put myself out there, to give my followers a look into my real life, from the baby-food-smeared kitchen shots to the red carpet glamour shots. In the beginning, I was naive, I admit. I never imagined that people could be so hurtful to each other. I thought there were some unspoken rules of engagement that governed how we all interfaced with each other online.

I was wrong. After posting pictures of my growing baby bump, I quickly received a handful of incredibly angry comments from several followers, mainly women. After years of being in a relationship with a celebrity whom the media follows obsessively, I had developed fairly thick skin, but I have to admit that these comments really stung. They certainly gave me ample chance to practice Living Clearly. The strong words written on this forum by total strangers knocked my character and my body; they questioned the depth and honesty of my marriage. At first, I was overcome with boiling rage when I would read these comments. I was absolutely consumed with an anger that seeped into every part of my body. My head would pound, and my throat and jaw would clench. I could feel the negativity pumping through my blood. But I knew that I would get sick if

I allowed these feelings to remain inside my body. So I turned to the principles. And after pulling back and gaining perspective, breathing deeply, feeling my feet firmly on the floor, and connecting to that place of calm equilibrium inside me once again, I was ready to let go. I let it go by reminding myself that those people and comments had nothing to do with who I actually am. They didn't know me, I didn't know them, and the negativity behind their cruel comments was not something that I needed to internalize.

To be clear, letting go does not mean giving up or giving in. I very rarely respond to the people who spew negative comments on my Instagram feed. I usually just delete and

When It's Time to Let Go

We are given numerous opportunities to practice Letting Go all day, every day—and we often do so unconsciously. But you can train your inner Letting Go alert system by paying close attention to what is happening in your body in any moment. For example, if someone cuts you off aggressively while driving, nearly causing you to lose control of your car, you'll probably experience a strong physical reaction. The stress of the situation will cause your heart to beat quickly; you may also feel rage toward the driver that manifests as a tight feeling in your throat or a heavy feeling in your belly. By bringing your attention to these sensations in your body, you can start to use them as signals that you're smack in the middle of an opportunity to let go. In this case, you could follow through with the rage by yelling obscenities out your window or speeding up so you're on the driver's tail—or you could move through the first four Principles to get a sense of how you would feel if you followed through on your anger. You'd see that spewing curse words isn't representative of who you really are and leaves you feeling childish and empty, and that speeding up angrily just contributes to a sense of feeling unsafe while driving. Once you've taken some conscious breaths, found your seat firmly under you, and clicked into a calm sense of equilibrium (a process that can take place in mere seconds) you will be ready and able to let go. Letting go of your rage (or bitterness, disappointment, or regret, the list goes on and on) frees you from the grip of that emotion—notice how your body feels after letting go—and gives you space to connect to another human being's experience. You are no longer possessed by what has happened to you; you can see beyond that singular experience and into the possibilities of the future.

block the user, but every once in a while, I take a picture of the biting comment and post it as an image on my feed for all of my followers to see. I view these moments as teaching opportunities for the negative commenter as well as for the rest of the community, because I know that it doesn't just happen to me. This is my way of saying, "Hey, I'm a person, too!" while also reminding everyone that commenting on Instagram is not like sending someone a private e-mail; it is a very public forum. After posting two negative comments as photos, the amount of hurtful comments I received went down significantly. I think bullies often like to bully everyone. You can release the boiling sensation that a strong feeling can bring up in your body without losing your integrity; you can let go while still standing up for yourself.

TRUSTING WILL HELP YOU LET GO

Letting go has a relaxed feel to it, a gentle and receptive tenor, but one of the reasons it's so challenging is that there is also a leap of faith inherent in each moment. When we surrender, whether to the reality of what's happening in our lives or to the floor in Pigeon Pose, we take our hands off the steering wheel and trust that we will be held firmly or led confidently to where we need to go. We experience this risk every time we let go, even when we let go of old habits. There is a question connected to each moment of letting go: *Will I be okay if I don't pick up a cookie when I'm feeling sad? What will happen to me if I don't smoke a cigarette when I'm worried? How will I feel if I change my morning or evening routine?*

We are creatures of habit, and there is comfort even in harmful behaviors that we engage in consistently. Your regular late-afternoon brownie and Frappuccino isn't just feeding an addictive sugar craving, it has become an emotional place of comfort and safety, where you go when your workday becomes too challenging or boring or what you turn to if you're dissatisfied in another area of your life. It's basically a highly caloric security blanket. But I challenge you to ask yourself, *What will happen if I put the blanket down?* You will be okay. I promise.

It takes courage to let go of a safe routine and walk into the unknown. The key is to start slow, to prove to yourself that you won't die if you don't have your usual two glasses of wine when you get home from work. You need to see that your heart won't burst out of your chest if you don't soothe its loneliness with a sugary treat. You may feel the longing for the wine or the sugar bright and hot within you, and you may have to exert genuine strength to redirect all of that supercharged craving energy into something else—talking to a loved one, taking a walk, jumping up and down until the craving passes, or journaling. But you will see that you are more powerful than you imagined, that you are bigger than your cravings and your habits, and that the emotionally charged eating or drinking is simply covering up an issue or feeling that wants to be addressed directly.

Margaret is my poster child for courageous habit breaking. When we first met, she was a sweet and giggly woman in her midfifties and a regular in my group classes. She'd often come with her adult daughter, and though she was significantly overweight, she'd happily move through even the most challenging sequences. After a few months, she came up to me and asked if I was taking any more private clients. She was really enjoying

Rest Is the Best

Letting go consistently helps us factor in a necessary part of a healthy and vibrant lifestyle: rest. Without concentrated periods of restoration, it is impossible to sustain the fast-paced, ridiculously demanding lifestyles that most of us have today. Proper rest also enables us to work more efficiently and effectively. Without rest, we become depleted and unable to accomplish all that we hope to do.

I learned the very hard way that a life without rest is like a life without food or water; it doesn't work. The longer you deprioritize rest, the faster you hurdle toward a breakdown, physically or emotionally. Resting is not a luxury. It's not indulgent or selfish. In my family, I've made sure that slowing down is an ingrained part of our routine. Alec and I are extremely hard workers, our natural way is to push until we've accomplished what we set out to do, but I make sure that we have daily moments of strategic nothingness. This can look like a slow stroll to a local park with our kids, cuddling in bed together, or lots of giggling. Resting doesn't necessarily mean closing your eyes and sinking into deep sleep. It simply means breaking out of the go-go-go pace of your everyday life to actually feel yourself in your body or to check in with your loved ones. For an easy recharge, you can move into any of the poses in this chapter for 5, 10, 20 minutes or more. You will emerge refreshed and ready to take on what's next.

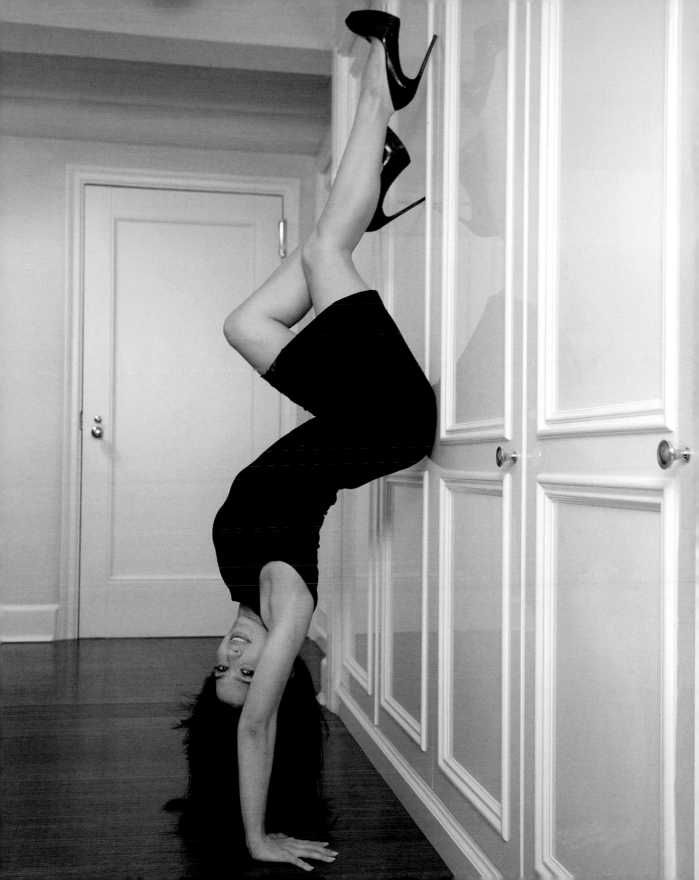

the group classes but was hoping that individual work would help to specifically address her weight. She told me that she wasn't always heavy and that her body had changed dramatically after menopause even though she exercised regularly. I agreed to work with her one-on-one.

Margaret seemed genuinely perplexed about the source of her weight challenges. I had my suspicions, so as soon as we began working together, I had her start a food journal. After a few weeks, we went over what she had captured, and the mystery was solved. Margaret and her husband, Paul, are lifelong New Yorkers—hardworking with stressful jobs—and use cooking and eating delicious food as a way to connect with each other and decompress from their jobs. Her journal revealed that highly caloric meals and a die-hard attachment to sugary coffee drinks (Margaret's morning routine) and lots of wine—they would drink a bottle at every dinner—were crushing her weight-loss goals. I helped her see that her portions at each meal were unnecessarily large and pointed out simple ways to get more nutritional value out of what she was eating.

> You can turn to any one of the principles at any moment to find your center.

She was open to making changes in her diet, but there were two places she refused to budge: coffee and wine. The beverages had starring roles as the opening and closing acts of each day, and she didn't want to live without them. So we focused on food. Margaret and Paul started making small changes in their diets and quickly saw results. They began making quinoa and beautiful pieces of fish instead of their usual heavy meals. And I guided her through navigating the menus at her favorite restaurants, teaching her simple hacks for making her prized dishes a little healthier.

The weight started rolling off, but she eventually hit a plateau. At that point, I asked her to look at what would happen if she didn't drink wine at dinner every night. She didn't have to cut it out entirely, but what if she decreased it to every other night or three times a week? She seemed genuinely open to this exploration; I felt her steely grip loosening on this established way of doing things. She and her husband limited their drinking at dinner, and her weight continued to melt away. Empowered by this incredible weight loss, Margaret then turned toward her coffee habit. I had her ask, *What would happen if I didn't drink a mocha every morning?* She started slowly, decreasing her mocha consumption to a few days a week, and as the weight continued to roll off—she was also maintaining her exercise routines and practicing yoga with me several days a week—she felt brave enough to try something new. Paul started making her green tea each morning. They made a ritual out of drinking unsweetened, dairy-free tea together, and she found herself looking forward to the time they would share before starting the day.

Margaret needed to know that drinking green tea with Paul would leave her satisfied and that she would be okay with a new way of doing things. She would not turn into dust or break into pieces if she didn't drink a mocha in the morning. Instead of being pulled along blindly by the tick-tick-tick of an established habit, she put herself back in control. She realized that a healthy body was more important than the momentary satisfaction that came from giving in to a craving or the perpetuation of an established routine, and instead she turned her energy to treating her body thoughtfully. In fact, she became so inspired by losing weight that she put tons of energy into learning how to make delicious, healthy meals and working out more often. Being healthy became her new habit. Margaret eventually lost 80 pounds, and she is still going strong today.

Here, at the end of the journey through the Living Clearly Principles, you are now prepared to navigate any challenging situation that comes across your path. You can turn to any one of the principles at any moment to find your center, to decrease stress and anxiety, to tap into your inner knowing and wisdom, or to stay the course of a health-and-wellness goal. As you move into the next chapters of the book, you'll see that the Five Principles will accompany you along your journey to a reimagined relationship with the food you eat and the way you work out. They will be your rock-solid support team, there to usher you through doubt or uncertainty, to remind you that you have more than what it takes to get where you want to go. I believe in you!

YOGA FOR LETTING GO

This sequence asks you to work, yes, but the primary focus is on letting go. This is often the hardest task of all. Ask yourself: How deeply can I sink into each pose? How much can I soften and release? Can I be selective about the effort I put into each pose? Can I learn to do as little as possible in order to rejuvenate and find calm? Throughout the sequence, pay specific attention to your breath; every exhalation is an opportunity to drop any tension you may be holding. *Approximately 15 minutes*

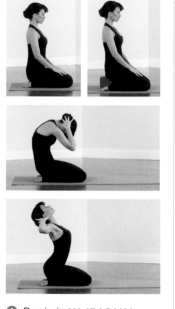

1 Begin in **VAJRASANA**, sitting back on your heels (you can always use a blanket or block to sit up on). Interlace your hands behind the base of your skull. As you exhale, round your spine, bringing your elbows together and tucking your chin. Inhale open up toward the ceiling, bringing your elbows wide and your chin up, taking a slight back bend. Exhale round your spine, looking down toward your belly button. Inhale look up, arching your back with your elbows wide. Exhale tuck and curl, rounding your spine. Inhale open up. Exhale close, releasing through the back of your neck. Take 10 rounds of breath.

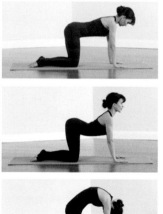

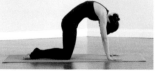

2 Come onto all fours, moving into **CAT COW**. Inhale arch your back into **COW**. Exhale round your spine coming into **CAT**. Take five rounds of breath.

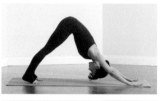

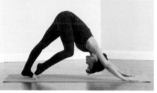

3 Inhale transition into neutral spine. Exhale come into **DOWNWARD FACING DOG**. Peddle your feet from right to left, waking up the backs of your legs. (The idea is to focus on places where you hold a lot of tension, creating movement in them and expecting release.) Take five rounds of breath, expanding with the inhalation and letting go with the exhalation.

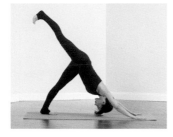

4 Inhale your right leg up **DOWNWARD FACING DOG SPLIT**.

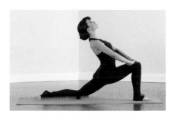

Exhale, step your foot between your hands, drop your back knee down to your mat, and inhale into **LOW CRESCENT POSE**, taking your hands to your front leg. Untuck your back toes (if this is too intense for your back knee, you can fold up your mat under your knee or use a blanket). Exhale bring your pelvis forward to feel a deep stretch in the front of your left hip (the psoas/hip flexors). Take five rounds of breath.

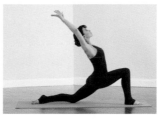

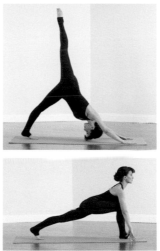

5 Inhale, hook your thumbs, and raise your hands above your head. Exhale your hands to the floor, framing the front foot. Inhale tuck your back toes under and transition into **DOWNWARD FACING DOG SPLIT**. Exhale open your hip up. Inhale extend your leg long, squaring off your hips. Exhale step your right foot between your hands. Inhale look forward with a strong back leg.

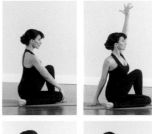

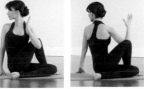

6 Exhale pop your left knee behind your right ankle and sit down for **SEATED SPINAL TWIST**. Inhale place your right hand behind your body next to your tailbone while reaching your left arm above your head. Exhale twist to the right, hooking your left elbow to the outside of your right thigh. With every inhale, relax your shoulders and lift through your spine. With every exhale, twist more deeply into the pose. Take five rounds of breath. Inhale, unravel, coming to face the center. Exhale counter twist in the opposite direction. Inhale come back to the center.

(continued)

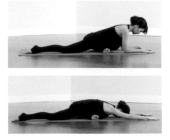

7 Exhale swing your right leg behind you into **PIGEON POSE** on the left side. Bring your left knee over to the left side of the mat, squaring off your hips and lengthening your right leg long behind you. (You can always place a blanket or block under the left hip or under the hip flexor of your right leg for support. This will prevent your body from tensing up, creating the ideal balance between challenge and ease, which leads to greater release.) Exhale release down. *Note:* As soon as you've settled in a pose, it's natural to think about what's coming next. But staying in intense poses gives you an opportunity to think about what parts of your body you are using and what parts you are able to release. In **PIGEON**, the shoulders and the glutes often get tight, and it's common to tense the back leg and the face. Remember, every single inhale gives you a chance to expand and notice tension and every exhale allows you to release.

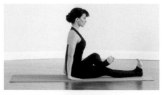

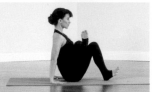

If the pose is too challenging, you can sit on your butt, extending your right leg long and butterflying your left leg open, crossing your left ankle just above your right knee, bending forward if that is available to you.

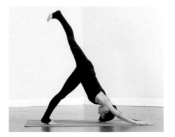

8 Press the floor away, remove props, and inhale into **DOWNWARD FACING DOG SPLIT** with your left leg up. Exhale open your hip up, regaining mobility and any circulation that was lost in **PIGEON POSE**.

Repeat the sequence on your left side, ending in Downward Facing Dog Split with your right leg raised. Bring your leg back down into Downward Facing Dog.

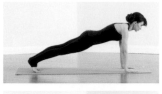

1 Inhale, transition your shoulders forward, coming into **PLANK POSE**. Exhale. Bend your **KNEES**, **CHEST**, **CHIN** to the mat.

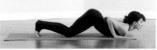

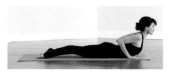

2 Inhale **BABY COBRA**.

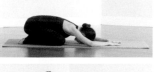

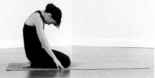

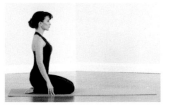

3 Exhale **CHILD'S POSE**, moving your sit bones toward your heels, forehead on the floor. Activate your navel toward your back, and very slowly begin to roll up your spine, tucking your chin, with your head slacking last.

4 Inhale your shoulders forward and up. Exhale them back and down. Take three rounds of breath.

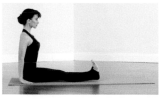

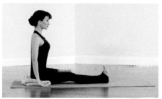

5 Bring your legs in front of you, flex your feet, and come into **STAFF POSE**. (You can always sit up on a blanket or towel or block, especially if you can't sit up straight and your lower back is rounded.)

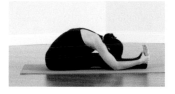

Take a deep breath in, and on the exhale, start to walk your fingertips toward your feet into **SEATED FORWARD FOLD**. (We have an obsession in our culture with touching our toes. If you need to touch your toes, you can always bend your knees and get to them easily, but if you're

reaching for your toes and you don't have that flexibility, your shoulders are going to come up toward your ears, which is a literal pain in the neck and the opposite of letting go. You want to keep your shoulder blades attached to your spine and your neck soft.) Take 10 rounds of breath. Inhale sit up.

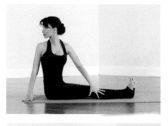

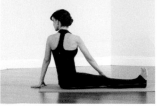

Exhale twist to the right. Inhale to the center. Exhale twist to the left.

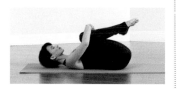

6 Release all the way onto your back and move into **APANASANA**, bringing your knees into your chest, wrapping your arms around your legs, and giving yourself a hug. This is a relaxing pose that releases a lot of tension from the body.

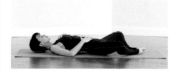

7 Place your fleet on the floor, butterfly your knees open, and press the soles of your feet together in **SUPTA BADDHA KONASANA**. Take one hand to your heart and one to your belly. Spend 60 seconds here releasing and letting go.

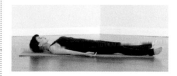

8 Move into **SAVASANA**, releasing everything to the floor. Stay here for as long as you like, focusing mind and body on letting go.

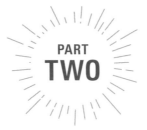

PART
TWO

FOOD & FITNESS

Do you treat your body well?
When it comes to eating and exercising, do you make the best choices you could?
Do you feel that you are worth it?

In Part One, you discovered ways of becoming present and improving how you relate to yourself, other people, and the world at large.

Now, it is time to use this knowledge to improve the ways you treat your body through food and fitness. These two things are vitally important to Living Clearly: The food you consume greatly contributes to how alert and capable you feel in body and mind, and exercising is one of the most immediate ways to clear the cobwebs in your head and really get into your body.

It's amazing when you start to notice how what you consume can instantly enhance and sustain your vitality and well-being or make you feel cloudy, dulled, and all fogged up. And how not moving for hours or days can put you in a slump and make everything seem gray. It's equally amazing how simple it can be to start to reverse that with modest shifts that truly add up.

When you feel good in your body, it's easier to stay present to yourself and life around you. Why? The mind wanders because it is seeking satisfaction. When you eat well and exercise regularly, your mind finds that the sensations in the body are more wonderful than anything else. Eating an energizing meal or sweating and strengthening and elongating your muscles—these create exciting and uplifting sensations, or sometimes peaceful and serene ones. It feels good inside! This draws the mind to stay present, and with mind and body working as a team, you feel awake and integrated.

But eating poorly or getting too sedentary creates a negative experience. Now the sensations inside the body are uncomfortable, awkward, or disappointing. The mind will jump to anything else—Twitter feeds, gossip chats, reality TV—to dodge that discomfort and get out of the misery. It quickly becomes hard to break free of these distractions and change course by, say, making a big salad or going to the gym. Sometimes you unconsciously amplify this shut-down state by using numbing behaviors and habits, like eating food that makes you more sluggish, drinking alcohol that sedates you, or losing yourself in gaming, partying, and even meditating (yes, this truly healthy practice can be abused if you use it to check out and escape from being in your body).

Don't think of food and fitness as two gigantic subjects that you have to master to be healthy. They go together. I've always considered eating to account for 80 percent of the healthy-body equation. If you put good things into your body in reasonable amounts, you won't have to log hours on the treadmill to burn them off!

Today, there is so much health news coming at us at all times, from scientific research to fad diets and workouts that guarantee a transformed body in 20 days, to experts with the secrets that will help create a new you, to lists of dos and don'ts for every bite you put in your mouth. It's dizzying!

I believe in simplifying the process right down to two things: Get clear on your relationship with eating and exercising using the Five Principles, and then have some dependable tools that you can turn to throughout the week—quick and easy meals that use whole-food ingredients, plus time-saving and effective exercise strategies that fit into your life. These small healthy steps can be powerful, and when put together, they pack a punch. Eating shouldn't be so complicated.

My experience is that with time, these simple approaches bring a special glow to your life—the glow that comes when you are digesting food well, are absorbing great nutrients and lots of water, and are at peace with your body. It comes when there's less struggle in how you treat yourself and good habits are successfully laid down. That's when you start to say, "I like where I've arrived, and I don't want to go back!"

This self-compassion and self-respect is the core of treating yourself well. When you wake that up inside, even if you're just starting on the path, you really do radiate health and beauty from the inside out.

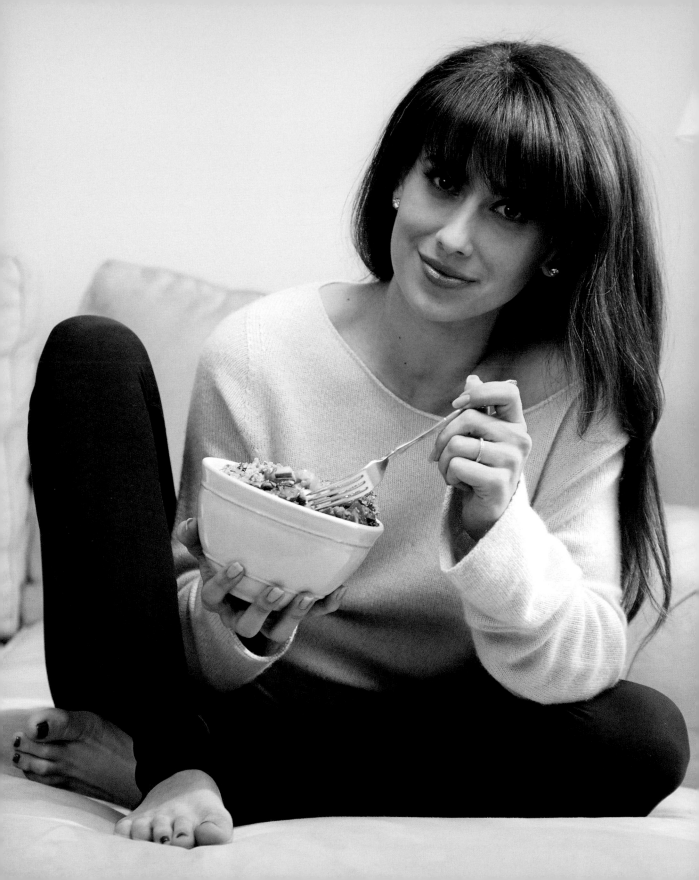

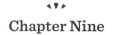

Chapter Nine

EATING CLEARLY

IT IS ASTONISHING HOW SOMETHING AS STRAIGHTFORWARD AS EATING can cause such drama and struggle in our lives. In all my years of teaching, I have yet to find one person who has always had a completely healthy relationship with food. This should come as some comfort if you struggle in any way with eating as well as you could. You are not alone, I assure you!

It took me years to develop a clear and healthy relationship with eating. For so long, I got it all wrong. Eating healthfully and enjoying the whole process of cooking didn't come easily to me. When it comes to food, I've lived lots of questions, and I've lived my way to the answers.

When I was 5 years old, I came home from my first sleepover and announced to my family that I had become a vegetarian. As a little kid, I had never equated meat with animals, assuming that eating food called "beef" or "pork" was the same as consuming an apple or a bowl of rice. But my friend's family was briefly trying out vegetarianism, and they had spent our evening together laying out the harsh facts about animals killed for meat and asking me questions like: *If you love animals, then how can you eat them?* I remember feeling horrified at the thought of my beloved furry friends getting slaughtered simply to end up on my dinner plate.

Vegetarianism was not as popular then as it is now, and very few resources existed to coach such a dramatic dietary transformation. With no familiarity or understanding of the changes I asked for, my parents questioned if I could get the proper nutrition to grow up strong on a plant-based diet. Also, as both worked grueling hours, where would they find the time to make two meals? And, perhaps most importantly, how could they afford it? They responded to my announcement by telling me that, as a child, my body was not mine to choose how to nourish and that everyone ate meat so I should, too. I will never forget the sternness in their voices as they labeled me powerless in the matter and commanded me to eat whatever they put in front of me.

Night after night, they gave me my carnivorous dinner, and I responded in my innate headstrong fashion: I wouldn't consume a single bite. This went on for quite a while, until my parents began to worry. They did research and found this bizarre substance called "tofu" that they subsequently bought, sliced off in slabs, and served to me raw every night with either ketchup or soy sauce. I ate this for years. Delicious it was not, too much soy it definitely was, but I happily consumed it day after day, knowing that no animals were harmed in the process.

Looking back, part of my intense desire to give up meat was for my love of animals, but if I'm being honest, it was also linked to what I was dealing with emotionally at the time. It was the beginning of an eating disorder that would plague me for the next 20 years.

As a teenager immersed in the world of dance, I became a master at depriving myself. Abusing my body through bingeing and purging became a way of life. When I moved to New York as a college student and a dance teacher, living on my own in the big city, eating consumed my thoughts. On the surface, it was about staying thin; at a deeper level, it was a method of numbing out the questions I didn't want to hear: *Could I make it? Was I worthy of succeeding? Did I even like myself?*

I was so caught up in the details of rigidly controlling what I did or didn't eat that I was blind to how this was undermining my efforts to make a good life. Physically, I was so tired that I would fall asleep on the subway between classes. My fuel tank dropped to empty constantly, I would get colds all the time, and my skin, hair, and nails were dull and weak. Mentally, my head was spinning. I couldn't see it, but I was literally giving my power away to my eating disorder.

I knew that what I was doing was not good for me. Frequently, I'd correct course and begin to eat—but then I'd tip out of balance, eat too much at once, and hate the way my body felt. The cycle of denial would start again. The irony, of course, was that as I stepped into the role of yoga teacher, I was guiding others to be at home in their bodies, but I was very confused about how to kindly and smartly inhabit my own.

The process I developed for my yoga students is what saved me. As I committed to teaching my Five Principles, I began to take them off the mat in all areas of my life. As I began to be more present and grounded, I stopped running away from the things that I feared. This finally gave me the courage to turn toward my biggest area of challenge: eating. I began to practice yoga "on my plate." I let my awareness help me become present to the experience of eating instead of escaping from it.

As I ate, I engaged some of my perspective exercises. Instead of doing muscular activating and releasing, I activated strong sensations of taste: a spicy-hot kick of pepper, a rush of wasabi, a waft of mysterious turmeric. This trick kept my mind engaged and interested in the food on my plate instead of obsessing about how to work off the calories and spiraling into judgmental and self-abusing thoughts. I looked up from the moment to see the broader perspective and connect to my goals. I wanted to resolve my food issues so that I would not pass them on to the children I longed to have in the years to come. I wanted to stay present while eating so I wouldn't check out and could experience the amazing blessing it is to eat.

I breathed intentionally as I prepared and ate meals to create a softer and more accepting state. I got grounded and settled into my body to wake up my capacity to feel what my body really needed. When I found my center—the seat of my will and courage—I was able to face my demons. I finally could feel that it was time to let go of the negative and sabotaging thoughts about food making me fat or somehow not okay.

After years of struggle, the clouds and confusion in my mind began to part. I remember coming to a realization that changed everything: *My body is smart, my body*

> I began to practice yoga "on my plate." I let my awareness help me become present to the experience of eating instead of escaping from it.

works, there is nothing wrong with my body. So I don't need to trounce it with weird diets and strict-sounding rules. I'm just going to listen to my body, be present while I eat, use common sense and a little nutrition education—and I'm going to go from there. Because all the worrying is driving me crazy!

◂▾▸

I was still in my early twenties when I began to take back my power around food. The task meant retraining myself to eat well, meal by meal. Being a penny-pinching yoga teacher, a vegetarian, and a type A achiever working crazy hours actually worked in my favor: I needed cheap, healthy, and fast, so I figured out systems for cooking simply and healthfully using affordable, whole-foods ingredients like bulk-bought grains and root vegetables. I taught myself to get enough protein through beans, quinoa, tempeh, and nuts—adapting my plate to what felt good in the moment and becoming more flexible about my eating "identity."

I had loved to cook since I learned in my family's kitchen, but for the first time, I was preparing food specifically thinking about how it would nourish me. When I ate out, I paid attention to the ingredients that made my meals delicious and expanded my repertoire of ingredients with shakers of seaweed, nutritional yeast, and jars of sunflower seeds. These vegetarian staples delivered a broad spectrum of essential minerals and vitamins and dashes of savory flavor, making simple things super tasty. And I discovered the essential missing element for looking and feeling great: fat! I needed good-quality, unprocessed fats for good energy, hormone health, and a balanced brain and mood state. Bottles of extra virgin olive oil, jars of coconut oil, avocados, and nut milks and butters became my best friends.

I also cut ties with some things that didn't serve me. Listening to my body, I noticed how dairy foods made my chronic asthma worse. I let milk products go entirely, and I found I no longer needed an inhaler; I breathed better and felt happier and less congested in my system.

The more this way of eating became ingrained, the more my body thanked me. I got back to a healthy weight, my energy levels—so critical to sustaining my long working hours—elevated, my immune system strengthened, my hair became shinier and stopped breaking, my skin became clear and bright. And as a result, I loved my body much more than I had before. I was also much more accepting of its quirks and respectful of its

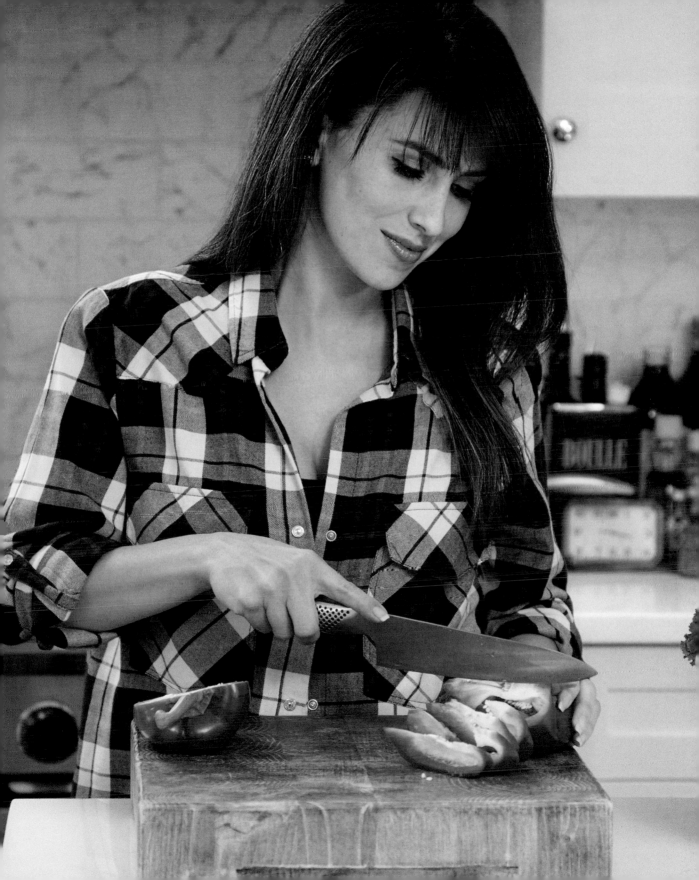

needs—and less rigid and fearful about what eating certain foods would do to it. This softening brought joy to eating instead of the misery I'd experienced for so long. I had finally come home to my body.

I knew my relationship with food had truly been healed when, during my first pregnancy, I happily acquiesced to my doctor's request that I enrich my diet with eggs and fish. This may seem like a small thing, but for those who've struggled with control issues around food, it's not. Getting out of my narrowly defined comfort zone had always been painful for me, but suddenly it was exciting to change my meals to serve my body's and my baby's needs, and it was awe inspiring to watch my belly grow.

By becoming present to eating, I finally found the self-control I'd been seeking. It came from a calmer and kinder place of self-knowing and from listening to physical signals I had always ignored or overruled, like noticing true hunger and paying attention to how food felt, not just when I ate it but afterward, as well.

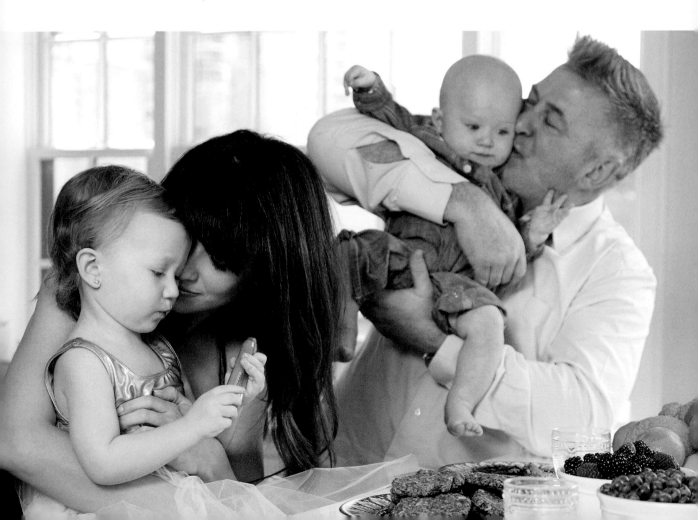

Noticing the impact that one day's worth of meals has on your sleep that night or on your strength, energy, and mood will give you objective information about what your body needs. It is like having a map to follow—simple and clear. This will help you take the reins back and chart an easy and permanent path forward, using food the right way, to power and support the life you want to live.

◂▾▸

This simple and wholesome way of eating is still the basis of how I cook for myself and my family today. I have a fairly simple and repeatable system in the kitchen. I use the same basic pantry ingredients, like quinoa and grains and beans of all kinds, in many types of meals. I concoct nourishing bowls of cooked grains and roasted vegetables that I store in the fridge and then customize from day to day with layers of cooked greens and a protein and toppings like hummus and delicious dressings. These make for a great lunch. In the morning, the bowl concept gets a breakfast twist: I mix oatmeal and granola with fruit, almond milk, and nut butter, or I take the quinoa I've premade and turn it into the strange-sounding but amazing Zucchini Bread Quinoa Bowl (page 180). At night, it's about lentil and vegetable soups, baked fish, my vegetarian Shepherd's Pie (page 203), or my Pasta Primavera with Tofu (page 196) that we share as a family— or simple fare like stir-fries or my Stuffed Peppers (page 202) when my husband and I eat together later without the kids (which we make sure to do at least twice a week).

> Having a routine helps me stay on track. When there's food ready to go, I'm less likely to skip meals or get so hungry that I turn to impulse eating.

Having a routine helps me stay on track. When there's food ready to go, I'm less likely to skip meals or get so hungry that I turn to impulse eating. It makes the process of dishing up meals during busy days—with a vocal toddler at my heel and baby on my hip—much less stressful. And it means that on nights when Alec and I eat out or go to events—which often offers unpredictable nutrition—I have had good food all day and can go with the flow a little more. Sound hard? With practice you will get it. It is like adding all the right ingredients in a recipe. In the recipe section that follows, I'll share some tips and strategies for creating the routine in your kitchen.

My style of eating is basically this: Eat real foods! Whole foods like whole grains, fresh vegetables, unprocessed oils, beans, legumes, nuts, seeds, and fruits haven't been broken down, tampered with, or turned into boxed and packaged foods. They are ingredients that your body knows how to deal with. Your cells can read the information in this food and do their jobs!

Don't think that this whole-foods approach is about eating minimally or frugally. It's the opposite; it's about putting nutrient-rich foods into your body that fuel you with energy, deliver the physical building blocks of growth and repair, and even help you heal where you are out of balance. When you eat this way, you are using food for its true purpose: to sustain your body and feed your brain so that you can live your best life.

In case you're wondering, this way of eating is for everyone, not just vegetarians and vegans. Though I don't personally eat meat or dairy products, both can certainly fit into this eating style (and the recipes that follow will offer some ideas for doing this). What I've found is that by eating "mostly plants" (to paraphrase Michael Pollan, one of my favorite food writers), it is more affordable to buy quality ingredients, since organic or grass-fed meats and dairy products tend to be the priciest things in your shopping cart.

LAYING A FOUNDATION

Instead of focusing on taking things *out* of your diet, make it a goal to gradually add a few different things *in*. Broaden your scope to include more good foods (they will nudge out the bad ones!). This is a much kinder way to increase health and beauty. I avoid "do not eat" lists and strict demands that you exclude all sorts of foods from your diet; there are so many "right" ways to eat, so many variations in taste, geography, genetics, beliefs, and budgets. How could there possibly be one-size-fits-all?

Laying down a good foundation also gives you resiliency, so you can relax and have some fun. Because let's be honest, sometimes the thing that tempts your taste buds is completely devoid of any nutrition. My particular temptation is the straight-from-the-oven cornbread that's served at an old-school New York restaurant that Alec and I go to when the people we're eating with are not down for kelp noodles and kale. There is nothing healthy about this cornbread. It's got gluten, sugar, salt, and probably GMO corn, too, all wrapped up in one fluffy slice of goodness. But it is to die for! I order it with the salmon plate, and I savor every last bite. Since my baseline is strong, I know my body can

POCO A POCO/LITTLE BY LITTLE

Instead of trying to change everything you eat, keep it manageable. Just try one new thing this week. Make a dinner of my Vegetable and Quinoa "Paella" (page 200) instead of your normal pasta and cheese; try a bowl for lunch instead of a tuna sandwich. If you're packing food for your children, send them to school with Muffin Pan Mushroom and Spinach Frittatas (page 179) in their lunch boxes or a green smoothie in their thermoses for snack time. Some of these dishes can be made in bulk and frozen for the future. The idea is not to have to cook fresh every single day (few of us have time for that). Some days, it could be as simple as applying a piece of advice from The Five Big Ideas section (page 141) to one of your meals that day, like adding a big serving of spinach when you might otherwise forget. The more you do one new thing each week, the more you build a foundation of healthy eating without necessarily doing a radical overhaul.

handle it. I call this strategy "keeping my cup near empty." With a diet of nourishing, unprocessed foods as my daily norm, a few drops of fun food once in a while won't make my cup of health spill over. My body can accommodate the occasional splurges, and I don't stress or feel guilty one bit because I know I'm not rocking the boat.

There are times, though, when the cup runs so full that there is no room for playing around. Even a few drops will push you to overflowing. When I met Alec, his cup was close to the brim. After years of eating out, eating late, and eating too much, he'd fallen into some bad habits without realizing it. His sugar intake was far too high, not just due to sweet foods and white carbs, but to pasta, sauces with hidden sugars, and snacks. We'd only just started dating, so this was a little awkward. I quietly watched what he ate, only mentally jotting down my secret wish list of what I'd tell him if he asked.

One day, his doctor told him his blood sugar was at prediabetic levels and he had to make changes—immediately. This was an alarming wake-up call that rocked him to the core. He called me and asked what to do. I readily gave him all of the thoughts and advice I had been collecting through watching him eat for months. His cup was so full that his body couldn't metabolize even a bite or two of sugar without causing insulin disruption, and this was leading him dangerously close to a chronic disease. To counter this as quickly as possible, he followed a strict regime: Pasta, bread, and any refined carbohydrate were out; all sauces (including his beloved sweet-and-sour Chinese sauce, a sugar-fest) were out; and even all fruits were nixed except for small servings of very-low-sugar berries. (I actually recall telling him, as he spooned more of that sweet sauce on his plate, "It's a sauce, not a soup!")

This was a moment for drastically putting order where disorder had taken over; his body chemistry couldn't rebalance until the aggravating foods and drinks were removed. We began eating all our meals together following these stricter parameters and exercising together daily. Gradually, his body chemistry reverted to normal, his blood levels normalized, and he lost a lot of weight, as well! This episode completely changed his relationship to eating. By hitting a crisis point, he gained a new perspective on some of the unhelpful habits that had become his normal without his realizing it, like eating his major meal of the day late in the evening when it's harder to digest, and usually doing it in a social setting, where it's much harder to exercise restraint.

I share this story because it's important to know that what may be quite harmless for some people can be poison for others. If I eat sugary cornbread occasionally, it is fairly benign; for someone who's got insulin issues, it is poison. There are moments to be slow and steady with dietary changes, and there are moments to take swift action! And sometimes, complete vigilance is required throughout your life because even small amounts of the wrong thing irritates or inflames you. Getting to this level of awareness of food sensitivities can require some fine-tuning work, and this is much easier to do if you have the basic foundation of clear eating down already.

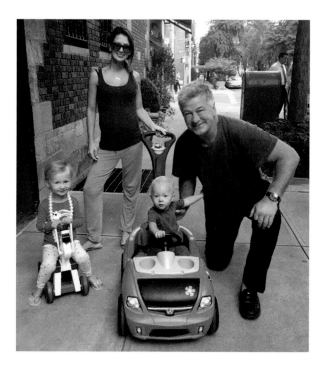

THE FIVE BIG IDEAS

These simple and broad guidelines for eating clearly—feeling nourished, sustained, and sharp—help make any diet healthier. They can boost the way you function, feel, and look, and you can incorporate them whether you eat meat or not or whether you already follow certain dietary protocols for your unique needs.

❶ Choose Quality

Even if you eat very healthfully, you're likely deficient in some nutrients. The way our food is farmed and produced today leaves a lot of gaps in our nutrition, undermining our foundation of health. My philosophy is to keep it "real" (lots of whole foods and fresh produce), cook as many of your own meals as you can, and always get the best ingredients you can afford because they will deliver the highest nutritional value to every cell in your body. This way of eating doesn't have to be pricey. Stock up on produce at farmers' markets; get bulk-size pantry items (beans, legumes, grains) from health food stores and co-ops; and find deals online for fats, oils, nuts, and seeds and ship them to your door. All this puts quality foods in your pantry and fridge while saving a little money for better-quality eggs, meat, fish, and dairy products if you eat them.

> *Organic is a big word in my household. It still costs more than conventional—though this is changing by the year. One cost-saving strategy is to check out the "Dirty Dozen Plus" (a list that is easily found online) for the foods that have the highest pesticide load when farmed conventionally. Make them your priority when buying organic.*

Applying perspective helps here. You can feed yourself and your family food that is cheaper and more convenient to prepare, but you will likely eat a lot more of it because the food itself won't make you feel as full as nutrient- and fiber-packed ingredients would. And don't discount how the real cost will come later when it impacts your health. Plus, getting more nutrition out of your meals is actually more about spending time than money; after all, homemade lentil soup is as cheap as it comes.

Tip: Many farmers' markets offer fresh, pesticide-free produce that is not certified organic because it's expensive and hard for small producers to get the certification. By asking around, you can find "nearly organic" produce at very good prices.

For meat, dairy, eggs, and fish, the most nutrient-rich choices, if you can afford them, are grass-fed meat and dairy above grain-fed; pasture-raised eggs or, secondly, organic eggs above regular; and wild fish above farm-raised. Some cheaper cheats? Get canned fish—like sardines, mackerel, herring, and salmon—into your pantry. They are less gourmet than fresh fish but an incredible way to get protein and essential omega-3 fatty acids into your diet. Frozen vegetables and fruits retain many of their nutrients as they are usually picked and flash frozen ripe. Ideally, get organic if you can.

When buying packaged goods—nut butters, nut milks, cereals, and healthy snacks—look for products containing the fewest ingredients, with names you actually recognize and with nothing extraneous or artificial added. Make sure they have the lowest sugar content you can find. Reading every word on the label only takes a few extra seconds.

❷ Green Your Plate

We all know that eating fresh vegetables and fruits at every meal is good for us. They infuse us with a rainbow of vitamins, minerals, and phytonutrients with powerful protective benefits, as well as fiber. But that doesn't mean we always do it! All that information can go in one ear and out the other. A small side serving of lettuce once a day just is not enough. Our bodies thrive on a lot more than that! The trick is to shift the way you see your plate.

Try relating to your leafy greens from a new point of view. Yogic texts say that fresh produce—raw and cooked—will bring more *prana*, or life energy, into your body. Just as plants deliver oxygen into the air, when eaten, they bring that same life force into you! I know that when my diet is full of leafy greens and other colorful vegetables, I feel clean, alive, at ease, proud of my body, and more mindful. So as you commit to consciously using your breath, it goes hand in hand to also eat more greens. Here's how:

- ▶ Substitute a big portion of steamed vegetables any time you'd normally have crackers, toast, or chips. Try going for cruciferous or leafy veggies most of the time: broccoli, cauliflower, bok choy, kale, chard, spinach.

- ▶ Prepare roasted squash, beets, and carrots where you might otherwise use white potatoes. Discover the spiralizer: a nifty gadget that peels vegetables into noodles that you can steam and use instead of pasta!

► Throw handfuls of spinach into a smoothie. This is a savior for my kids; they get their greens without any bribing or cajoling on my part. Before you know it, you'll be using greens and vegetables at every meal and in your snacks.

Once you get on a roll with this, it becomes a habit, something that makes food prep creative and fun. And the benefits of a plant-rich diet will start to sink in. There is so much to discover when you open nature's medicine chest.

Tip: If your plant-rich diet leans toward vegan, take care to include foods that are fortified with B_{12}, or take B_{12} supplements. This is an essential vitamin we cannot get from plant food alone. Adding nutritional yeast on savory dishes is a great way to add this in—it's used in many of my recipes—though if you eat exclusively vegan, you'll need more than this alone to be well.

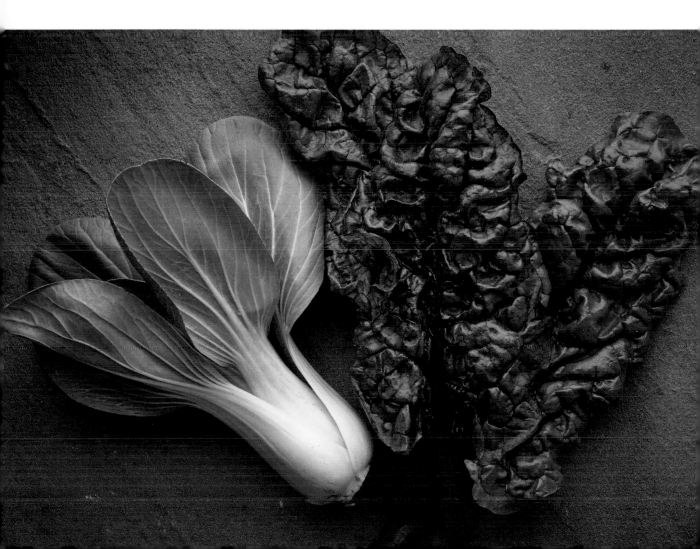

❸ Make Friends with Fat

The science is irrefutable: The low-fat fanaticism of the past was based on faulty thinking and pushed people to consume lots of carbohydrates instead. The problem is that eating refined carbohydrates and sugars in excess spikes insulin, and these foods get stored on the body as fat! The new science shows that *this* is what creates saturated fat in our blood (not eating butter or coconut oil!), wreaking havoc on our health. It's time to fall back in love with fat.

Every system in your body needs fat to function well—including your brain. Incorporating enough of the right fats into your diet will make a big difference in how grounded you feel and how clearly you think. They give you more energy per calorie than any other food, reduce hunger so you eat less, keep you warm, support a stable mood, and give you shiny hair, strong nails, and good skin, plus much more. Though some body types do well with more fats, and some do better with less, your lifestyle and activity level will also impact the amount that works for you. Bottom line: There is absolutely no reason to be scared of the letters *F*, *A*, and *T*!

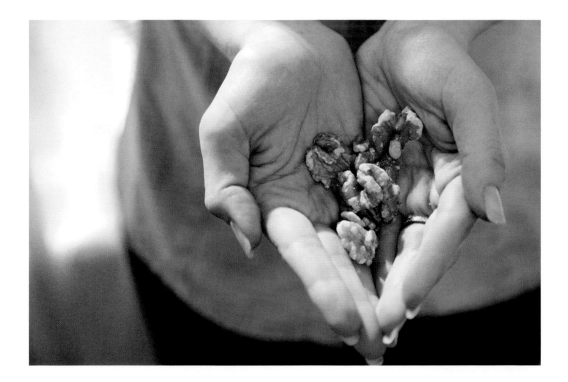

Let's keep it really simple: Eat fats as close to the way nature intended as possible. Use coconut, virgin olive, flaxseed, walnut, and avocado oils. Always pick expeller- and cold-pressed oils; they are unrefined and have not been treated with chemicals or solvents in processing.

If you eat meat, get it grass-fed if you can: It contains a healthy balance of omega-3 to omega-6 oils, which helps to maintain good health and prevent inflammation and disease.

Steer clear of oils like soy, canola, corn, cottonseed, and peanut. They cause inflammation and create heart disease. Know that most restaurants, most processed foods, and all fast foods use these oils—yet another reason to cook your own meals. Whatever you do, nix the partially hydrogenated oils—aka the dreaded trans fats—which are directly linked to obesity, heart attacks, and cancer. Though these are being phased out of all foods, they still exist, especially in the cheapest baked goods and snack foods, fast foods, and butter-type spreads.

As you get to know your body well, you'll start to figure out how much fat you need. But it's fairly simple: When you eat real food and don't overdo anything, your body stays happy.

4 Sugar, Fixed

It's not that sweet foods are all bad; it's that we've completely lost our perspective on them. In nature, sweet foods like berries or honey are the occasional but delectable treat for the body as they are seasonal or hard to find. Today, sugary foods are available everywhere, all the time, and they are made up of completely unnatural ingredients that our bodies cannot use—like high-fructose corn syrup. It's in savory foods, in condiments (yes, ketchup!), and, worst of all, in drinks (sodas are literally liquid sugars).

My technique when I get the itch for sweets is to eat strong, dark chocolate. It hits the spot and kicks the sugar craving out of my body. If you've got a sugar habit you want to drop, try cutting all the sweet treats from your diet entirely except for two pieces of dark chocolate in the afternoon (or at night if it doesn't keep you up). If you don't like dark chocolate, try a (small) date or dried fig—nature's best candy. Under these limitations, you will look forward to it and find it more satisfying. And you will lose weight. Plus, having sweetish healthy snacks in your repertoire will gradually change your palate. My healthy whole grain pancakes (page 182) smeared with almond butter will satisfy the urge for sweet while giving you protein and fat to quiet the cravings your body is having. These strategies work for my toddler when she craves a cupcake; they can totally work for you!

If you don't have a battle with sugar cravings, then as long as your cup stays pretty empty, enjoy and seduce your senses with special treats—especially when shared with people you love. Make these treats occasional and good quality, and make them deliberate (when you're choosing to indulge with the full awareness that it's for the purpose of pleasure, then there's nothing to regret). For me, it's coconut ice cream or a magdalena pastry—a treat that makes me smile and remember that life is sweet.

❺ Nix the Tricky Snacks

My nephew, who was raised macrobiotic, used to call junk food "tricky foods"—things that look, smell, and taste like food but are actually horrible for your body. The crunch of orange-coated corn chips, the snap of Ritz crackers (with their high-fructose corn syrup), the rustle of bagged popcorn coated with trans fats—this world of impulse eating is scarily man-made and artificially enhanced. They "trick" you.

Apply some perspective, and you might see how corporations have designed these foods scientifically to light up your pleasure centers with unnaturally big flavors. They give instant gratification when you're bored, restless, or seeking distraction. Get present when you reach for them, and you may realize that when you're eating these things, you're almost never truly hungry. You're looking for something missing—a feeling, a sensation, a moment of satisfaction. You'll notice how they don't satisfy you; they leave you craving *more* because they are full of chemicals that the body cannot process and that merely trick it into feeling fed. Having that awareness is a little triumph and the start of letting them go!

But how do you physically ditch the habit?

The more you fill your diet with a diverse array of tastes and textures from good ingredients, the less interesting those fake-food sensations become. Your palate shifts: Natural flavors start to register as appealing while overly bold, phony flavors become garish to your mouth. Know that savory snacks often hook you in by satisfying your need for crunch and by using MSG and other synthetic ingredients that capture the sweet-salty-sour taste that chefs call umami. Ditching tricky foods becomes totally doable when you combine your own savory flavors and satisfy your senses. A crunchy rice cake topped with tahini and a sprinkle of nutritional yeast or a smear of miso paste gives the same umami flavor, as does flax crackers topped with avocado and tangy cheese (if you eat dairy) or a dash of nutritional yeast, which vegans often substitute for Parmesan.

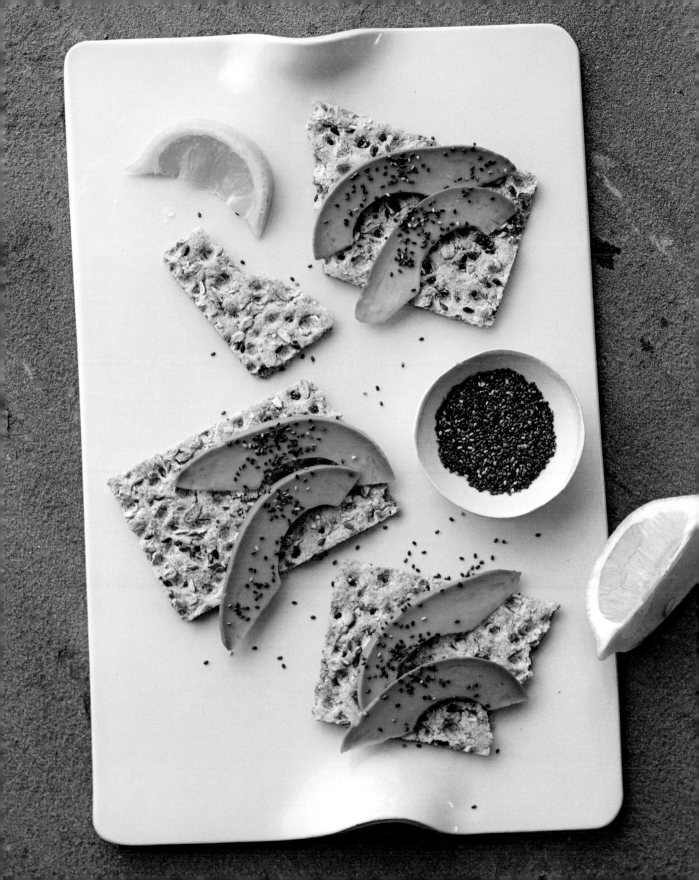

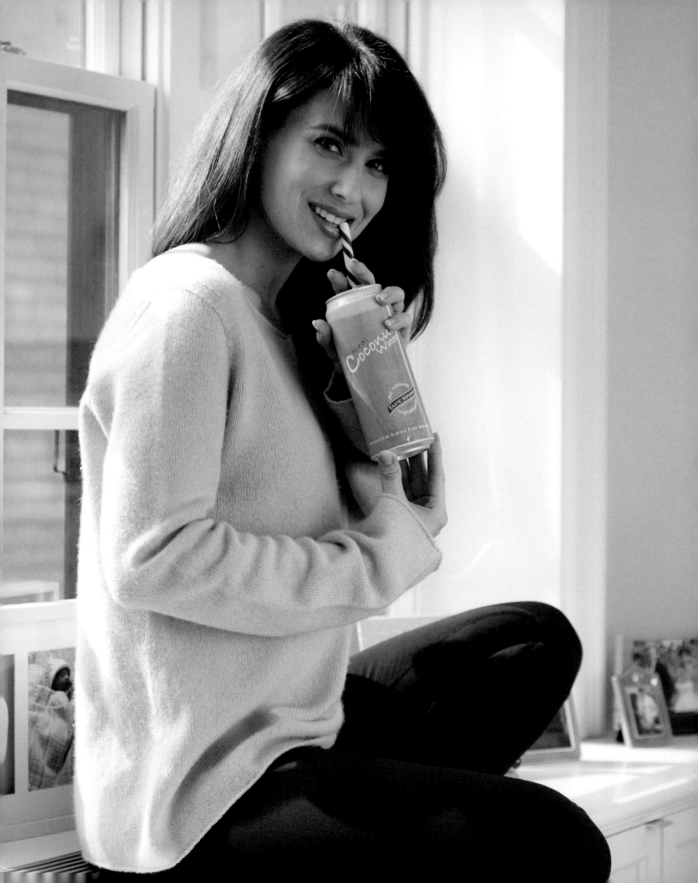

6 ... And Don't Forget #6: Hydrate!

Drinking plenty of water is critical for flushing toxins out of the system and for regulating blood pressure, and it also helps to moderate hunger. Often when you think you are hungry, your body is actually asking for water. Try hydrating first, and then ask how hungry you are again. There's no need to drink like a maniac; we also get water from raw vegetables, fruits, soups, and smoothies. When I'm breastfeeding, I use a secret weapon to stay hydrated: coconut water in the morning and evening. Compare the sugar content of different brands before you buy, however, as it can vary widely.

Start experimenting with these Big Ideas today. Know that dietary changes can take an initial period of being really strong, so make sure to use the Five Principles guidelines that follow to keep yourself on track. The good news is that your body does want to eat this way! Soon you will be craving a healthy diet and itching to start an exercise plan alongside it. It's like getting over caffeine. It sucks for a few days to a week, but then you feel reborn.

TIPS FOR STAYING ON TRACK WHEN EATING OUT

Here are a few of my road-tested ways for eating clearly and sticking to your goals when ordering off a menu.

- At a sushi restaurant, ask for a naruto roll, which uses cucumber or radish in place of rice.

- Just say no to the bread basket, and order burgers wrapped in iceberg lettuce to avoid the white-flour bun.

- Ask for dressing on the side so you can regulate the amount. If you don't know what the dressing is, choose olive oil and balsamic vinegar (to avoid bad fats).

- To avoid the risk of your entrée being cooked with bad fats, ask for it to be cooked in olive oil.

- If you feel pressured to eat something that's not serving you, you can always say that you have an allergy to it.

YOGA ON YOUR PLATE: USING THE FIVE PRINCIPLES TO BUILD A HEALTHY RELATIONSHIP WITH FOOD

Why can't I lose weight? Why can't I stick to my resolutions? Why can't I break my snacking habit?

When you become present to the act of eating, you start to see what really drives your actions—stress, emotional upset, boredom, habit—and find the space to make a different choice.

Turn to the Five Principles to help make the shifts you seek. They are practical tools for connecting thinking with feeling so that you are more present to the experience of eating, noticing the sensations in your body *and* the thoughts and emotions in your mind. This is essential if you want to break the pull of cravings, curb snacking and overeating, and ultimately take back your power around eating. I use them all the time, mainly to keep myself on track when I get wrapped up in work and time flies by. I breathe to slow down, ground to get back into my body and listen to its needs, and balance to make sure I am well fed. Practicing being present creates a shift in your relationship with food. You begin to make choices deliberately and learn to feel confident about them. Here are common challenges that the Five Principles will help you meet in a new way.

THE CHALLENGES: *Gripped by cravings or struggling to choose the healthy option or to control portions*

THE PRINCIPLE: *Perspective*

Applying perspective helps to insert more space into a charged moment of hunger or desire to allow you to make a deliberate choice. It lets you see beyond the moment of instant gratification to the bigger picture of consequences. When the urge to sink your teeth into a doughnut or pour that second glass of wine is overwhelming or you're exhausted after a long day and just want to *eat right now*—chicken in a bucket is good enough!—clicking in to perspective can alter the course of events.

Food is not just an in-the-mouth experience: *Will I like this? Will it taste good? Will I feel happy when I eat it?* It's a whole-body experience. Activate perspective to visualize the food moving through your entire body—from your mouth, through your throat, into your digestive tract, into your bloodstream, to your liver for processing and separating out toxins for your kidneys or intestines to deal with, and then into your cells to be used as energy or building blocks for new cells. Whew! In that new light, how does the high-fructose corn syrup, triple shot of espresso, or 28 grams of sugar per serving look?

Run through the four-step Perspective Process when the waiter comes to take your order or you are roaming the aisles of the supermarket (or raiding your refrigerator!). It is a powerful way to step back from automatic habits and make a different choice.

1. Pause. Wait. Notice an opportunity opening to change an impulsive behavior.

2. Zoom out to the bigger viewpoint. Ask: *How will I feel after eating this? How will I feel tomorrow?* Consider the impact on your energy and mood, how your digestive system will handle it, or how your sleep may be affected by it. You might even check in with how your self-esteem or looks will fare—blemishes, circles under the eyes. This step also applies to skipping meals or eating too little. Denying yourself good nutrition will also have physical and mental consequences.

    Then zoom out further: *If I do this repeatedly, how will I look, feel, and function in a year, or 5 years from now?* Perspective is the realm of the mind that loves to dive into the past and speculate about the future. Harness it now to imagine the outcomes.

3. Reframe with a question: Is this food or drink serving a purpose? Is it feeding true hunger or supplying quality nutrients to your body? Or is it your chosen temptation that you're going to enjoy to the max? Get clear on why you're eating what you're eating. If you're under the grip of cravings and munchies, this step empowers you to see them, name them, and decide whether to serve them. Finally, if you decide it's necessary, you can . . .

4. Make a different choice.

    If you tend to overeat, activating perspective can help break a habit that may stem from your childhood, when adults forced you to finish your plate. Pause, pull back, and remind yourself that you can eat a little now, then a little later. Perspective helps you look down the line and see that another meal will come soon.

Eating Impact Log

Keeping a food log is a time-tested way to gain clarity on which foods help you and which ones hurt. It doesn't require complex calorie counting, unless you want that. Record brief notes about what you eat and drink throughout a day, and note how you feel later that day, that night, and the next morning. Note your energy levels, your mood and mental clarity, your sleep quality, your digestion and elimination patterns (bowel movements), and any physical and mental effects and symptoms.

For example:

- ▶ 2 cups of coffee midmorning; feel jittery and agitated all afternoon
- ▶ Extra-dark chocolate late at night; wired, couldn't sleep
- ▶ Pasta at dinner; headache in the morning
- ▶ Skipped lunch; couldn't concentrate, had cravings

After a few days, see if patterns emerge between certain foods and certain symptoms. Armed with data, it's a little easier to drop an old habit and try something new.

THE CHALLENGES: *Rushing through meals, not digesting well, feeling overly anxious about eating*

THE PRINCIPLE: *Breathing*

When you're rushing around trying to fit eating into a hectic day, the first thing to go is your breath; it gets short and constricted. But improper breathing creates a stress response, which makes you feel anxious. And feeling unsettled or nervous around eating makes you more likely to reach for something that pacifies you (like sweet foods or comfort foods) rather than nourishes you. Worse, if you're under chronic stress, elevated cortisol levels can cause you to gain fat. This is why it is so important to initiate calm and steady breathing during and after a meal. It switches on the relaxation response, which not only frees you of anxious feelings but also frees up energy for digestion and promotes circulation. As you breathe fully, you deliver more oxygen to feed the "fire" of digestion in your belly, your metabolism increases, and you break down your food more smoothly.

Cooking with Calm

Don't forget to tend to your breath while you tend to the stove. My friend and recipe collaborator Melissa Petitto says that if she's ever in a bad mood while cooking, she leaves the kitchen to take some deep breaths and settle down before coming back so that her presence while making food for others is calm and kind. Cooking is an opportunity to put love and care into your body and the bodies of those you love. Are you stressed, or are you content? I want the food I cook to make my family's life better, and remembering to breathe helps me stay true to that, even when time is short and my hectic household doesn't feel very namaste.

Check in with your breath when mealtime approaches or when you notice you are hungry. Is it shallow? Is your belly tight? If so, initiate a fuller breath. Try initiating Sama Vritti (page 68). It helps you to slow down so that you take a moment to feel into what would best serve your body in this moment. Relaxing helps to loosen the grip of a craving or habit and give you the reins over your choices again.

Practice taking steady, relaxed breaths during and after a meal (talking less while eating will help!). This feels forced at first, but eventually it becomes second nature. And it is a tool you have at your fingertips. Steady breathing as your meal digests is a powerful shift that you can do starting today.

THE CHALLENGES: *Eating too much, never feeling complete, persistent snacking*
THE PRINCIPLE: *Grounding*

Reading news on smartphones over lunch, whipping through e-mails with a latte in hand, lunching while driving—it's amazing how out-of-body we can be when we eat. We spend so many of our meals in our heads. This isn't just a wasted opportunity to savor tasty sensations. Eastern sciences say being in a heady, thought-filled state when eating creates toxicity in the digestive system and dullness and fatigue. To get the maximum vitality from food, you must eat in a settled and grounded state.

Take a break from mealtime multitasking for a day. Commit to sitting quietly with your meal and *not* reading, talking, or making plans for what you need to do next. Instead, notice the sensations in your body—the feel of your body on the chair and your feet on the floor, the sensation of chewing and the burst of flavors in your mouth, your posture as you sit and eat. Get into the feeling of being in the body before you eat. If you're waiting in line to pick up lunch, practice getting grounded by doing the Relevé exercise from page 90.

Ask yourself: *Am I aware of my body as I eat? Do I feel settled and rooted? How often does my mind leave my plate and get caught up in thoughts?* Play with bringing your mind back each time it wanders (which it will!).

From this grounded state, you can start to notice the moment in the meal when you are *nearly* satisfied. This helps you make a conscious choice to stop before you are absolutely full—even if there is still food on your plate. Ending your meal when you are 70 percent satiated is a classic trick for ensuring you don't overload your digestion since it takes a few minutes for everything you've consumed to really be felt. If this brings up

LEARNING TO OBSERVE

Knowing why you're eating is key to changing any unhelpful habits. Play this simple game: Tag some of the meals, snacks, and drinks on your Eating Impact Log with the reason you actually consumed them. Look especially for the nonessential ones. Be honest. The reasons could include: *I was hungry; I was bored; my brain needed a pick-me-up; I was sad; it looked delicious!* Don't judge the reasons; just notice them. This switches on the ability to observe eating from a neutral place and then decide, *How did it serve me?*

resistance, remember, there will be another mealtime quite soon. Use any remaining hunger to fuel your inspiration for the next meal (if you do this exercise, you might have leftovers to use, too).

When you find yourself itching for a snack between meals, get grounded again. Feel your body and listen to what it is really trying to tell you—that you're actually thirsty, that you want distraction from the task at hand, or perhaps that you do really need some nourishment. This helps you see if you're snacking from genuine hunger or just habit.

THE CHALLENGES: *Doubting your choices, swinging between extremes, fear of spiraling out of control*

THE PRINCIPLE: *Balance*

When you're in balance around eating, you feeling confident about your choices. You're clear on why you made them and relaxed about their impact. You pay attention, but you don't overthink or obsess about every bite; you have a sense of how much food your body needs, and you know most of what you eat is really healthy—some of it less so—and the overall effect is pretty good.

You also eat at the right time of day, and you have a plan for eating and know where your food is coming from, so you don't spiral into a cranky, low-blood-sugar state and eat impulsively.

There's a real pleasure in getting to this centered place. Eating starts to feel instinctual, and what you eat satisfies your needs. It's like when you have a bowl of steaming, chunky soup on a cold day or a vibrant tomato salad on a sultry summer night. The meal hits the spot: You feel nourished and well fed, with no cravings. This is eating clearly!

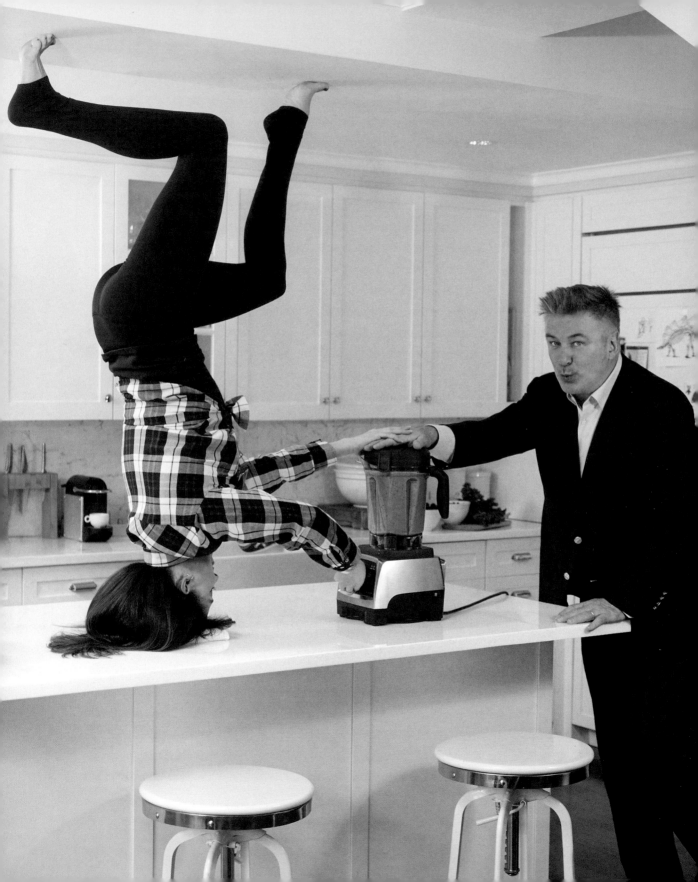

Try this mindful-eating exercise with a food that brings up challenging feelings—probably something indulgent, whether savory or sweet. It might be something you usually crave and feel guilty about eating afterward. (A chocolate lava cake would be a good one to use!) Breathe, get grounded, and savor one bite. Put the spoon or fork down and notice the taste, texture, and smell; notice the way it makes you feel and any emotions or memories it evokes. Continue to eat slowly and deliberately without distraction. Notice everything good and special about the experience, and consider why you enjoy it so. Also pay attention to how it affects your energy, mood, or clarity later on.

The next day, take a minute to breathe, ground yourself, and then revel in how much you enjoyed it! Apply some perspective about how that particular indulgence is a pure treat for your senses once in a while. Balance that with remembering any overstimulating sensations that didn't feel so good (like a head rush from too much of that chocolate

Letting Go of What Other People Think

Other people can feel threatened when you change your lifestyle. It highlights what they don't want to change in themselves. They prefer the "old" you—the one who hangs out and does what they do. Sometimes sarcasm or unsupportive comments come up and push you off your path. I know my husband got some of these when he ate strictly. There were some jokes and eye rolling about his saintly habits. This can hurt, but that's when you lean on the Five Principles for help. They'll keep you connected to your goals when you're feeling judged or pressured to eat in a way that you don't want to. Eating is for your own good. It has nothing to do with anyone else.

When these situations happen, turn inward for a second (people don't even have to realize you're doing it). Run through perspective, breathing, grounding, and especially balance. Connect to your will, the part of you who's sure of the reasons for your choices. Let other people's opinions and baggage around food go; they're not yours to own! And let this remind you to look for people who will support your goals—a friend you can call or meet with or an online community dedicated to healthy eating. Quick check-ins with people who get what you're doing will go a long way.

cake!). Own your choice and imprint the positive association in your memory. Remind yourself that there is no need to crave that food again today. Yesterday's experience was complete; perhaps one day in the near future you'll do it again. For now, you can move on without thinking much more about it or getting consumed by the experience.

If you've ever spiraled out of control around food—or lived in fear that you would—this awareness exercise builds the capacity to decide to be at ease and not struggle. It takes effort at first, but it builds muscle memory. Try the mindfulness exercise with increasingly mundane items. When you perform it around a cup of tea or a morning grapefruit, you'll know you've truly made progress in being present to your meals.

A chef was once asked how he restrained himself from overeating as he cooked and tasted things. He said, "You take the first bite to have the experience; the second bite to savor and hold on to the experience. With the third bite, you're just trying to re-create an experience that has already happened." When you are truly *in* the experience of eating, you might find that just one or two bites of something intensely flavored or rich will deliver plenty of sensation.

Balance involves making adjustments in how you manage your cooking and eating to find that stable center point where it all flows more easily.

Do you wait too long before eating in the morning, getting frazzled as a result? If so, alter the course: Stop skipping breakfast and eat something nourishing!

Do you eat your biggest meal at night, close to bedtime? Most healing arts in the world point to noon as the optimal time to eat big, protein-rich meals because your digestive fire burns brightest then, just like the sun. Adjust your meals and see how it feels.

Do you struggle to prepare food for the days ahead and always scramble at the last minute? This calls for revamping your system and taking time out to plan for the week ahead. Once you've shopped, start by making the fixings for my Living Clearly Bowls (page 165) and getting them in the fridge. They'll last several days and help you see how advance prep in the kitchen aids your quality of life.

THE CHALLENGE: *Being rigid or overly controlling or too serious about eating, wanting to give up a food or eating habit but feeling stuck*

THE PRINCIPLE: *Letting go*

Perspective, breathing, grounding, and balance help you become present to eating habits and discern which foods positively impact your body and moods. They also show you places where foods or habits aren't worth it.

This primes you to ask the question: *Could I let it go?*

This might include habitual patterns that don't actually serve you (like eating too much, not eating enough, or snacking unnecessarily) or specific foods that don't work for you. The more you become present, the harder it is to ignore or tolerate the ruts you are in. Asking yourself, *Could I let it go?* is a kind way to start getting out of them. It simply invites the possibility of living a different way.

TAKING THE FEAR OUT OF CHANGE

If improving your diet feels overwhelming, take these four basic concepts to heart.

▶ **Keep it simple.** You do not need to be a gourmet chef. What I eat might be kind of boring, but I love it because it is easy and I know how good I'll feel after each meal. And clean, simple ingredients have good flavor! Keeping it simple in the kitchen has been a powerful technique for getting my kids to develop a palate for clean and natural eating; it teaches them to enjoy the flavors of the actual ingredients without tons of stuff thrown on top.

▶ **Make it repeatable.** Get a repertoire of reliable healthy staples down, and then mix and match them. You're not looking for a wild adventure every time you eat; you just want to feel good.

▶ **Block out time.** Designate hours for prepping and cooking during the week and make them nonnegotiable. Make double portions of recipes when you cook to stock your freezer.

▶ **Keep at it.** We are creatures of habit. Over time, eating healthfully will become part of your daily routine, just like brushing your teeth or taking a shower.

Letting go may also mean letting go of rigidity and finding more joy in what you eat. Eating shouldn't become tedious or devoid of pleasure. It's not an execution. See what resistance comes up when you ask the question, *Could I let some of this strict control go?* Does your body tense or your breath shorten at the idea? Does your head buzz with reasons why not, and does your center become anxious and unbalanced? If you've found comfort by putting rules around the way you eat, these questions can be scary.

Breathe, ground, find your center, and ask the question again. Maybe you can't let it go right now. You're still living the questions. Just keep asking them while committing to eating clearly. One day, the answer will be maybe, and then, finally, yes. Part of the process of becoming present is letting go of control and trusting that by simply engaging with yourself in this new way, you are letting it all unfold. Using the Five Principles, you are developing mindful eating, so know that you will be okay if you stray! The worst thing that can happen from one daringly different meal is that you don't like it.

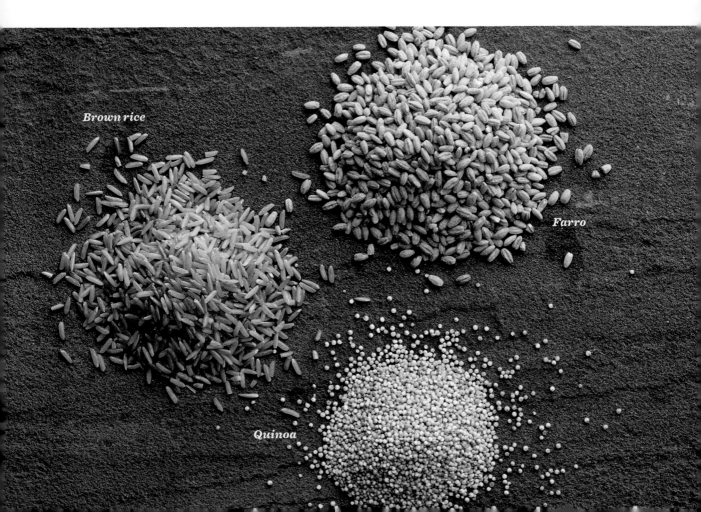

Brown rice

Farro

Quinoa

THE RECIPES

The recipes in this section are my go-tos—the staple meals and snacks I return to over and over again. They use simple, repeating ingredients and are meant to be doable in the busyness of life. And they are delicious! When friends come over, these are what I serve most often, and my kids eat most of them, sitting by our sides.

The kitchen is a very forgiving place. Not every meal has to be perfect. It just has to feed you with good ingredients! So play, experiment, and, above all, don't stress. With a few fresh, nutritious ingredients in your bowl, your meal will satisfy you, give you energy, and make you feel terrific.

THE LIVING CLEARLY PANTRY

Having a well stocked pantry and some must-haves in my freezer takes the pressure off eating well daily. I know that no matter how busy life gets, and even if I haven't had time to shop, I can always rustle up something simple, nourishing, and good.

You don't need all these ingredients to get started with the recipes that follow, but many are used several times.

GRAINS AND LEGUMES

An assortment of whole grains, like quinoa (all colors of it), brown rice and wild rice, rolled oats, amaranth, barley, bulgur, millet, farro, and teff. A few types of brown rice pastas and whole wheat pastas. A variety of lentils (red; green; and French, or "puy," lentils). A variety of beans (canned or dried), such as adzuki beans, black beans, and chickpeas.

NUTS, SEEDS, AND DRIED FRUIT

Almonds, cashews, pecans, walnuts, pepitas, and pine nuts. Flaxseed and chia seeds—ground or whole. Golden raisins, dried cranberries, dried apricots, and dates.

FLOURS, ALTERNATIVES, AND BAKING SUPPLIES

Gluten-free flour (though you could use whole wheat), almond flour, coconut sugar, wheat germ, olive oil spray or coconut oil spray for muffin pans and for making pancakes and waffles, cream of tartar, and coconut flakes.

SPICES, HERBS, EXTRACTS, AND FLAVORINGS

Cinnamon, nutmeg, cloves, ginger, safflower or saffron, dried oregano and basil, vanilla extract, chamomile tea, lavender extract, sea salt, and ground black pepper. Nutritional yeast, chili paste, tamari or reduced-sodium soy sauce, honey, and maple syrup.

OILS AND VINEGARS

Unrefined olive oil (for sautéing), extra virgin olive oil (for dressings), coconut oil, and toasted sesame oil. Balsamic vinegar, brown rice vinegar, white wine vinegar, and dry white wine.

MILK ALTERNATIVES

Canned coconut milk, full and reduced fat. Other nondairy milks, like almond, hemp, soy, and cashew.

SNACKS

Jars of almond butter and tahini (sesame seed butter) and rice crackers.

IN THE FREEZER

Frozen kale, spinach, blueberries, mango, and other fruits for smoothies, plus assorted frozen vegetables. And dark chocolate bark!

IN THE FRIDGE

Eggs, coconut yogurt, tofu, tempeh, hummus, and sprouted wraps are always in the fridge. Brown rice miso paste, olives, Dijon mustard, and a good bottle of zingy white albariño wine are usually in the fridge door.

Living Clearly Star Ingredients

These four staples of my recipes may be new to you but are well worth getting into your kitchen!

COCONUT PALM SUGAR—has a lower glycemic load than regular cane sugar with bonus trace minerals, too. It's a healthier sugar option that has a lovely caramel flavor. I use it in my carrot cake recipe and other treats.

NUTRITIONAL YEAST POWDER—gives a nutty, savory, cheesy flavor to all kinds of foods and can help mimic cheese sauces if you don't eat dairy. You'll find it used in several savory recipes.

PEPITAS—raw, shell-free pumpkin seeds are green in color and full of essential fatty acids and hard-to-get vitamin E and trace minerals. Used widely in Spanish cooking. I love to scatter them into all kinds of dishes and use them in a trail mix with dried fruits and nuts.

QUINOA—cooks like a grain but is actually a seed. It is full of good protein, fiber, magnesium, and more and is so adaptable. Always rinse it first in a sieve until the water runs clear. I use it in my bowls, my Shepherd's Pie, and even my pancake mix!

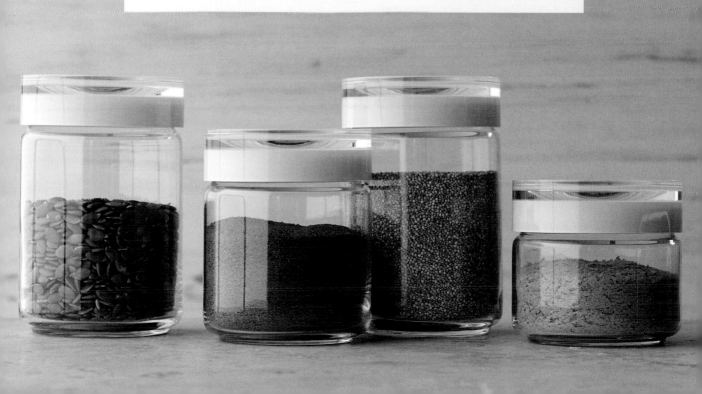

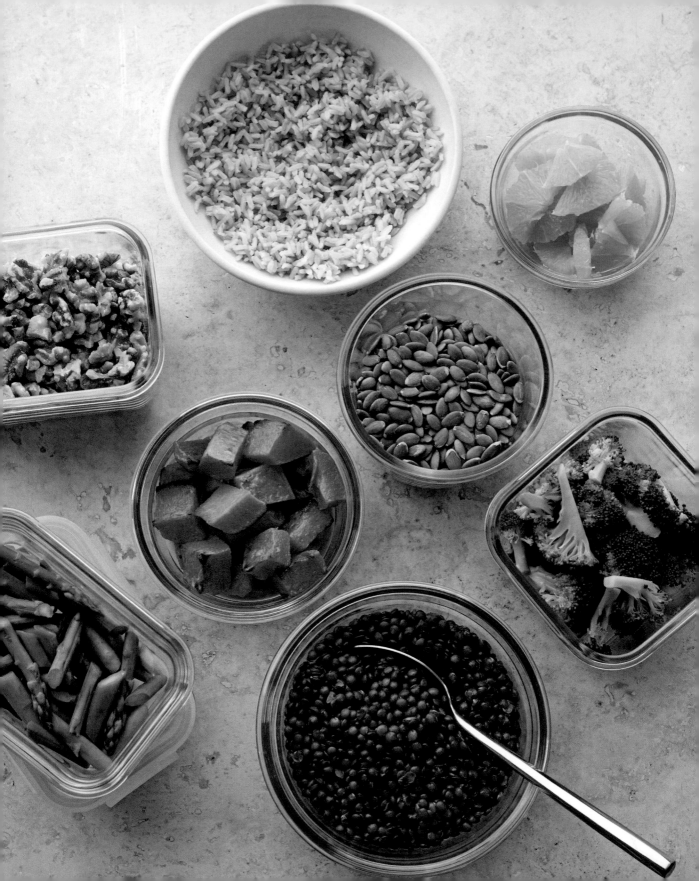

BUILD YOUR OWN BOWL

Perhaps the simplest way of eating healthfully is "the bowl." I use them for my lunch almost every single day. By prepping a few main ingredients—like grains, legumes, vegetables, and proteins—in advance, you make healthy eating systematic and simple. If your staples are ready to go, all you have to do is assemble and then decorate with your toppings of the day! You can customize your bowls in a thousand ways. The more nuts, seeds, and healthy condiments you get into your cupboards, the more fun you can have, making even a busy lunchtime a chance to savor satisfying tastes and textures.

Start by following this basic design:

1. A hearty base layer like grains or roasted root vegetables or a mix of both.

2. A generous serving of greens or other vegetables, cooked or raw.

3. Ideally, it has a protein of some kind—anything from tempeh to a hard-cooked egg to chicken, or you might like lentils, black beans, or a scoop of tasty hummus.

4. A little good fat; consider adding some avocado, one of my dressings (pages 174 to 176), or just splash on extra virgin olive oil.

5. Bump up the flavor and texture by experimenting with savory twists—a splash of tamari or a sprinkle of nutritional yeast, perhaps a scattering of pepitas or sunflower seeds or any other crunch. It's up to you!

You don't have to be exact, but the approximate proportions to make a satisfying and nourishing meal are:

---

1 cup cooked grain or root vegetable + 4 ounces protein (about the size of a deck of cards) or ½ cup cooked legumes + 3 cups raw vegetables or 1½ to 2 cups cooked vegetables + 1 tablespoon seeds or nuts (optional) + 1 serving dressing

---

Bowls can be eaten at room temperature or warmed up, depending on their components and on your mood that day. To warm, I put everything but the fats and flavorings in a steamer on the stove, warm lightly, transfer it scoop by scoop to my bowl, and then add the toppings and dressings. You can use a microwave if you prefer, but don't overdo it (90 seconds is plenty); it's not supposed to be piping hot.

LIVING CLEARLY BOWLS

I love the calming and centering effect of sitting down with a bowl. When I wrap my hands around one, I pause to take in the wholesome ingredients and I slow down, get anchored, and commit to nourishing myself well. Bowls switch on a mini mindful-eating experience!

I created one bowl for each of the Five Principles. Designed to delight the senses and satisfy the taste buds in very different ways, they are my best combinations yet! (Added bonus: Each of the dressing recipes can be used on a variety of salads and sides throughout the week.) Enjoy putting together these combinations—follow the approximate amount guidelines above and the cooking directions for each component that follow—and see if the qualities of each principle are conjured as you eat.

These particular bowls do not include proteins; add what you like, cooked simply (no need for a marinade here, the dressings deliver the flavor). It's a cinch to cook portions of grains and legumes that can sustain you for a few meals. The trick is getting the right ratios and cooking times, which are just a quick search on the Internet.

PERSPECTIVE

Spicy kicks of flavor and a rainbow of color and texture keep the mind engaged.

Grain + avocado + blueberries + raw spinach + sunflower seeds + Spicy Mustard Dressing (page 174)

BREATHING

A medley of aromas and flavors make a vibrant, energizing meal.

Grain + pumpkin + roasted garlic, onions, and Brussels sprouts + pepitas + Chili-Lime Dressing (page 174)

GROUNDING

Root vegetables—pulled from the earth—ground you with good sustenance.

Grain + root veggies + lentils + greens + Ginger-Carrot Dressing (page 175)

BALANCE

Adzuki beans, easy to digest and filled with nutrition, are balanced with an Asian-inspired dressing.

Grain + mushrooms + adzuki beans (or lima, kidney, chickpea, fava) + snow peas + broccoli + Tahini-Miso Dressing (page 175)

LETTING GO

This delicate, almost feminine bowl inspires a lighter hold on life.

Grain + asparagus + oranges + walnuts + Lavender, Chamomile, and Honey Dressing (page 176)

The Logistics

First, I make good-size portions of several components—a grain or two and some root vegetables—and store them in the fridge for the next 3 days. Sometimes I get really organized and cook some tempeh or fish in advance, as well. I use any tasty proteins from dinner the night before (the days when I discover a piece of roasted salmon with my name on it are the best!). Using canned beans is an option if you don't want to soak and cook beans (though make sure you are generous with your flavor if you use canned).

By playing with the idea, you will discover the combos you like best.

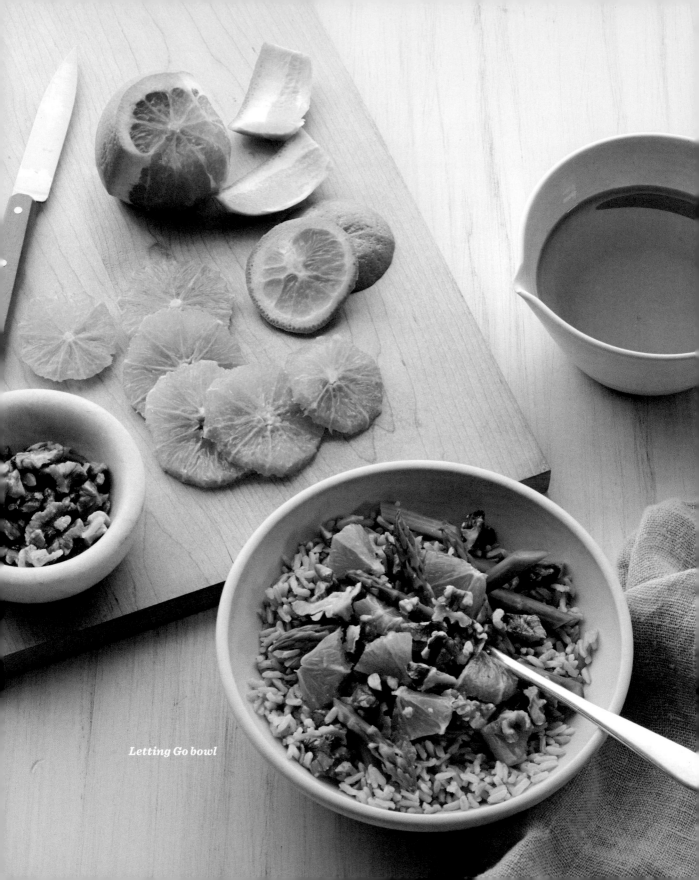

Letting Go bowl

COOKING INSTRUCTIONS FOR WINTER ROOT VEGETABLES AND SQUASH

Bake some root vegetables and squash each week and you'll have components of meals ready to go. Roasting creates caramelization and more flavor, so it's my go-to for squash. Use in bowls, as sides to entrées, or puree as a mash.

BAKING: Halve smaller squash (like acorn and delicata) and root vegetables (like parsnips, yams, and carrots). Scoop out the seeds if your vegetable of choice has them. Place vegetables on a parchment paper-lined baking sheet and top with a little olive oil, salt, and pepper. Bake at 350°F for 25 to 30 minutes, or until easily pierced with a fork. Add your favorite seasonings—such as ground cinnamon, paprika, ground cumin, garlic (chopped fresh, whole, or powder), or grated orange peel—to boost the flavor!

ROASTING: Halve squash (like acorn, butternut, and spaghetti). Scoop out the seeds. Rub the flesh side with olive oil or coconut oil, and season with salt and ground black pepper. Add any of your favorite spices and seasonings, such as paprika, dried rosemary, dried thyme, garlic (chopped fresh, whole, or powder), or orange juice. Flip the flesh side down and roast on a parchment paper-lined baking sheet at 400°F for 40 to 45 minutes, or until the skin is blistered and the flesh is tender. Insert a knife to test for doneness (the knife should go in and come out easily).

COOKING INSTRUCTIONS FOR OTHER VEGETABLES

You can quickly steam any vegetables you like just before using: spinach, Swiss chard, kale, zucchini, cauliflower, broccoli, asparagus, snow peas. Almost anything will work, though harder vegetables obviously need longer steam times.

When I have a little more time, my favorite way to cook greens is to braise them (see page 170). Fill a container with them to use in your bowls or as a side to entrées. They are also a component of my Shepherd's Pie (page 203). Use any cooking greens you want, and mix different kinds if you like; pick what's fresh and looks appealing. Lasts for up to 5 days in the refrigerator.

BRAISED GREENS

—— SERVES 4 ——

1 tablespoon olive oil

2–4 cloves garlic, minced

10 cups mixed greens, torn into bite-size pieces (try kale, Swiss chard, spinach, and mustard greens)

½ cup dry white wine

½ cup vegetable broth

1 In a large stockpot or Dutch oven over medium heat, warm the oil. Add the garlic and stir for 30 seconds.

2 Add the greens, wine, and broth and stir to combine. Cover, reduce the heat to medium-low, and cook, stirring occasionally, for 5 to 7 minutes, or until wilted.

BRUSSELS SPROUTS (BREATHING BOWL)

Toss with chopped onion and garlic and a little olive oil, salt, and pepper. Arrange in a single layer on a parchment paper-lined baking sheet and roast at 425°F for 20 to 25 minutes, stirring halfway through, or until crispy and caramelized.

ROASTED MUSHROOMS (BALANCE BOWL)

Slice and toss with a little olive oil, salt, and pepper. Arrange in a single layer on a parchment paper-lined baking sheet and roast at 425°F for 30 to 35 minutes, stirring halfway through, or until crispy and caramelized.

COOKING INSTRUCTIONS FOR PROTEINS

Here are some super-simple techniques for cooking proteins for your bowls, as well as for simple entrées and salads. The marinades listed on page 173 are optional but add a ton of flavor.

CHICKEN

1 Position a rack in the middle of the oven. Preheat the oven to 400°F. Line a baking dish with parchment paper, and rub it with 1 teaspoon olive oil.

2 Season 4- to 6-ounce chicken breasts with a little olive oil, salt, pepper, and other favorite seasonings. Place in the prepared baking dish.

3 Cover the chicken breasts with a piece of parchment paper and tuck the edges around the chicken.

4 Bake the chicken for 20 to 30 minutes, or until a thermometer inserted in the thickest portion registers 170°F and the juices run clear.

5 Let rest for 3 minutes before slicing, or cool completely and refrigerate for up to 1 week.

TOFU

1 Remove the tofu from its packaging and wrap in a clean dish towel. Weigh it down with something heavy, like a cast iron skillet or a large book, and press for 15 to 20 minutes. This removes the excess water from the tofu.

2 Cut the tofu into 1" cubes, thin slices, or sticks depending on how you plan to use it.

3 This step is optional but makes the tofu extra delicious! Whisk together your marinade of choice, and marinate the tofu in the fridge for at least 30 minutes or overnight if possible.

4 When ready to cook, preheat the oven to 400°F. Line a baking sheet with parchment paper and spray with olive oil spray or coat with 1 tablespoon olive oil.

5 Drain the marinade and pat the tofu dry. Arrange in a single layer, leaving space in between so that the tofu roasts and doesn't steam. Roast for 20 to 45 minutes depending on the cut of the tofu, or until the outside is golden and the pieces look puffed.

6 Eat immediately or cool completely and store in an airtight container for up to 1 week.

TEMPEH

1 Preheat the oven to 400°F. Line a baking sheet with parchment paper, and coat with olive oil spray or a little olive oil.

2 Tempeh, like tofu, is great marinated. Slice or cube and let it sit in your choice of marinades for 30 minutes to overnight. Remove from the marinade and place on the prepared baking sheet.

3 Roast for 15 to 20 minutes, or until browned and crispy.

4 Eat immediately or cool completely and store in an airtight container for up to 1 week.

FISH

1 Position a rack in the highest position of the oven. Preheat the oven to broil. Line a baking sheet with parchment paper, and coat with olive oil spray or olive oil.

2 Place the fish fillets (about 4 ounces each) on the prepared baking sheet (skin side down if they have skin).

3 Drizzle with a little olive oil, and sprinkle with salt, pepper, and any other flavors you wish (try paprika, tarragon, dill, or grated lemon peel).

4 Broil for 3 to 7 minutes depending on the thickness of the fillet or until the fish is opaque (salmon) or the fish flakes easily (other fish). The fish should be lightly browned on top (salmon should show a little whiteness on the sides from the fat).

5 Serve immediately or cool completely and store in an airtight container for up to 3 days.

FOOLPROOF HARD-COOKED EGGS

1 Place eggs* in a single layer at the bottom of a saucepan and cover with an inch of cold water. Add ½ teaspoon salt.

2 Bring the water to a boil over high heat. Turn the heat off, leave the pan on the burner, cover, and let sit for 10 to 12 minutes.

3 Strain the water and place the eggs into a bowl of ice water for 5 minutes.

4 Peel under running water.

5 Store in a covered container for up to 5 days in the fridge.

Older eggs peel easier than fresh eggs; 1 week old is perfect.

PROTEIN MARINADES

These quickly kick up the flavor of any type of protein—except for eggs! Though I typically use them on tofu and tempeh, try them with chicken breasts (marinate for 2 to 24 hours) or seafood (30 to 45 minutes). They make enough for four 4-ounce protein servings.

ASIAN

*3 cloves garlic, minced +
2 tablespoons fresh ginger, minced +
2 tablespoons tamari + 1 tablespoon
chili sauce + 1 tablespoon sesame oil*

DIJON-HERB

*3 cloves garlic, minced +
2 tablespoons Dijon mustard +
2 tablespoons chopped fresh herbs
(parsley, thyme, basil, tarragon, etc.) +
1 tablespoon olive oil*

LIME-CUMIN

*1 tablespoon grated lime peel + 1 clove
garlic, minced + 1 tablespoon olive oil
+ 1 teaspoon ground cumin +
1 teaspoon apple cider vinegar*

SPICE BLEND

*1 teaspoon ground cumin + 1 teaspoon
paprika + 1 teaspoon dried oregano +
1 teaspoon chili powder + 1 clove
garlic, minced + 1 tablespoon olive oil
+ 2 tablespoons sherry vinegar*

SPICY MUSTARD DRESSING
(Perspective)

—— MAKES ¾ CUP :: SERVING SIZE = 1 TABLESPOON ——

Whole grain mustard is so versatile, and in this peppy dressing, it packs a punch of flavor. Designed to play with the spinach, creamy avocado, and plump blueberries of the Perspective Bowl, it's also great on roasted salmon, so try adding that to the mix!

2 cloves garlic

⅓ cup whole grain spicy mustard

¼ cup white wine vinegar

¼ cup extra virgin olive oil

½ teaspoon salt

2 scallions, green and white parts, minced

In a blender, combine all the ingredients. Blend until smooth. The dressing can be stored in an airtight container in the refrigerator for up to 1½ weeks.

CHILI-LIME DRESSING
(Breathing)

—— MAKES ½ CUP :: SERVING SIZE = 1 TABLESPOON ——

I created this dressing almost by accident, and soon I was putting it on everything I ate. The tangy lime and spicy chili balanced with honey makes any bowl or salad really exciting!

1½ tablespoons grated lime peel

2 limes, juiced (about ½ cup)

1 clove garlic

2 tablespoons chili paste (such as sriracha)

1 tablespoon honey

1 tablespoon tamari or reduced-sodium soy sauce

¼ cup toasted sesame oil

In a blender, combine all the ingredients. Blend until smooth. The dressing can be stored in an airtight container in the refrigerator for up to 1 week.

GINGER-CARROT DRESSING
(Grounding)

—— MAKES 1 CUP :: SERVING SIZE = 2 TABLESPOONS ——

If you love the ginger-carrot dressings at Japanese restaurants, then try this! Spoon it on a mixed greens salad or roasted veggies, or try it with the Grounding Bowl.

2 large carrots, roughly chopped (about 2 cups)

4 tablespoons jarred minced ginger

1 clove garlic

¼ cup brown rice vinegar

¼ cup tamari or reduced-sodium soy sauce

2 tablespoons toasted sesame oil

1 tablespoon honey

In a blender, combine all the ingredients. Blend until smooth. The dressing can be stored in an airtight container in the refrigerator for 1 week.

TAHINI-MISO DRESSING
(Balance)

—— MAKES 1½ CUPS :: SERVING SIZE = 1 TABLESPOON —

Creamy, savory, and filled with satisfying umami flavor, this dressing is also a great dip for roasted and raw veggies. Drizzle it over grains or greens; miso's rich taste and tahini's smooth texture will make the simplest bowl deeply satisfying. Tahini is a great source of calcium, and miso is legendary for its healing properties.

½ cup tahini

¼ cup brown rice miso paste

½ cup water

1 clove garlic

2 tablespoons grated lemon peel

1 lemon, juiced (about ¼ cup)

In a blender, combine all the ingredients. Blend until smooth. The dressing can be stored in an airtight container in the refrigerator for up to 1 week.

LAVENDER, CHAMOMILE, AND HONEY DRESSING

(Letting Go)

—— MAKES 1⅓ CUPS :: SERVING SIZE = 2 TABLESPOONS ——

This dressing is such a surprise. It's super light, so think about pairing it with mild ingredients like quinoa and baby greens so it doesn't get overwhelmed. The aroma alone is something so special. Awaken your senses with this one, and inhale slowly before taking that first bite.

4 bags chamomile tea

1 cup boiling water

2 tablespoons honey

1 teaspoon lavender extract

3 tablespoons white wine vinegar

¼ cup extra virgin olive oil

½ teaspoon salt

¼–½ teaspoon ground black pepper

1 Combine the tea bags and water. Brew for 10 minutes. Remove the tea bags and discard.

2 In a blender, combine the tea and the remaining ingredients. Blend until smooth. The dressing can be stored in an airtight container in the refrigerator for up to 2 weeks.

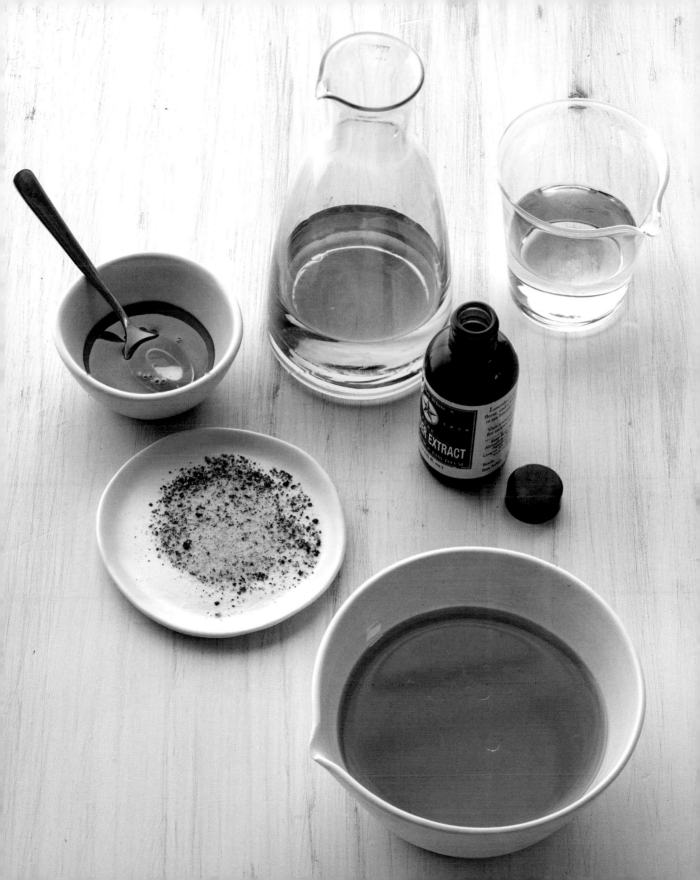

RECEIPES

MUFFIN PAN MUSHROOM AND SPINACH FRITTATAS

I love serving these tasty frittatas for brunch and then using leftovers as an easy lunch with salad the next day. Not only are they simple to make and store, but they also hook kids with their fun cupcake shape. Before they know it, they're munching on a protein-and greens-filled meal that will keep them going for quite a while.

1 tablespoon olive oil

1 small onion, diced (about 1½ cups)

2 cloves garlic, minced

1 package (12 ounces) frozen mushrooms

1 package (12 ounces) frozen mixed greens

6 large eggs

⅓ cup milk of your choice (soy, cashew, hemp, almond, dairy)

½ teaspoon salt

½ teaspoon ground black pepper

½ cup nutritional yeast or Parmesan cheese

1 Preheat the oven to 400°F. Coat a muffin pan with olive oil spray or coconut oil spray.

2 In a large nonstick skillet over medium heat, add the oil and onion and cook, stirring frequently, for 5 minutes, or until golden brown and wilted. Add the garlic and stir for 30 seconds.

3 Add the mushrooms and mixed greens and cook, stirring occasionally, for 5 minutes, or until the mixture is dry.

4 Divide the vegetable mixture among the prepared muffin cups.

5 In a medium bowl, whisk together the eggs, milk, salt, and pepper.

6 Divide the egg mixture among the muffin cups. Sprinkle the nutritional yeast or Parmesan on top of each muffin. Bake for 12 to 15 minutes, or until the centers of the frittatas are set.

7 These freeze wonderfully! Allow to cool completely and then store in an airtight container for up to 1 month in the freezer.

ZUCCHINI BREAD QUINOA BOWL

This flavorful and surprising alternative to oatmeal is a great way to use some of the cooked quinoa you've made for your lunch bowls. These are great reheated, so bake a bunch at a time and use them as an easy-to-grab breakfast on the go.

1½ cups packed grated zucchini (use the large-size cheese grater holes)

1 cup cooked quinoa

1½ teaspoons ground cinnamon, divided

¼ teaspoon ground nutmeg

¼ teaspoon salt

1 cup milk of your choice (soy, cashew, hemp, almond, dairy)

¼ cup ground chia seeds

¼ cup raisins

1 tablespoon vanilla extract

2 tablespoons coconut palm sugar or raw sugar

1 Preheat the oven to 450°F. Grease or spray four 1-cup ramekins with olive oil or coconut oil or line 4 large muffin cups with paper liners.

2 In a medium saucepan or pot over medium heat, cook the zucchini, quinoa, 1 teaspoon of the cinnamon, nutmeg, and salt, stirring frequently, for 2 to 3 minutes, or until the zucchini begins to soften.

3 Add the milk, chia seeds, and raisins. Increase the heat to medium-high and bring to a boil. Reduce the heat to low and simmer, stirring frequently, for 4 to 5 minutes, or until thick and bubbly.

4 Remove from the heat and stir in the vanilla.

5 In a small bowl, combine the sugar and the remaining ½ teaspoon cinnamon.

6 Scoop ¾ cup quinoa mixture into each prepared ramekin or muffin cup. Sprinkle with the cinnamon and sugar mixture. Bake for 15 minutes.

7 Allow to cool for 5 minutes and serve.

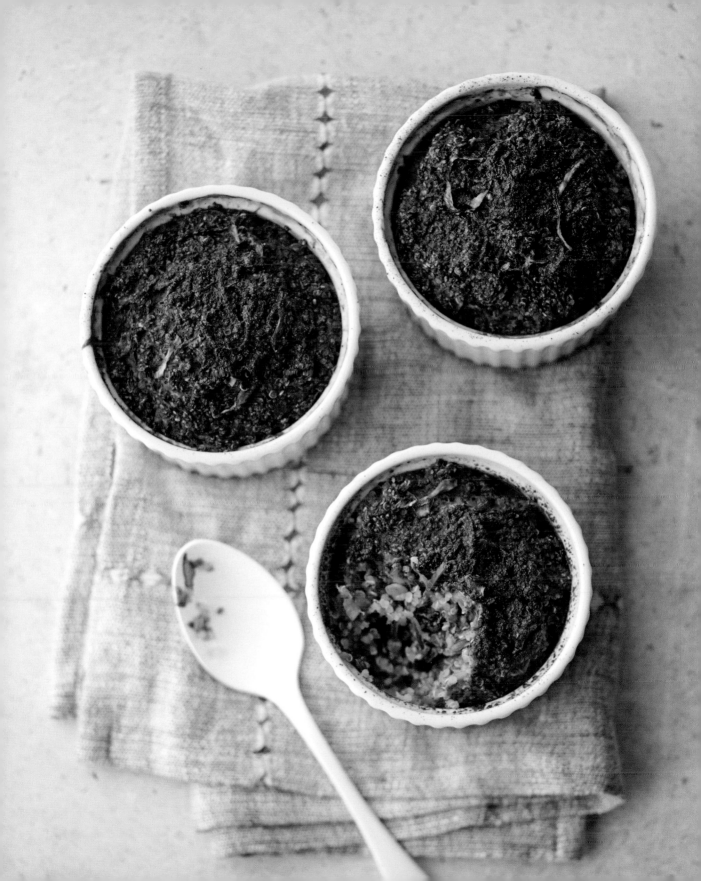

WHOLE GRAIN PANCAKE AND WAFFLE MIX

Who doesn't love a stack of pancakes or waffles? This recipe lets you feel good about feeding them to your family. With banana lending sweetness, you might not even want added sugar or maple syrup on top. In my house, we spoon fresh berries over them in the summer and cooked apples and pears in the fall and winter.

1 cup cooked quinoa

1 cup rolled oats

¼ cup wheat germ

1 tablespoon ground flaxseed (optional)

1 tablespoon baking powder

1 teaspoon ground cinnamon

½ teaspoon salt

½ cup milk of your choice (soy, cashew, hemp, almond, dairy) (increase milk to ¾ cup for waffle batter)

2 large ripe bananas or applesauce

2 tablespoons coconut oil or light olive oil

1 teaspoon vanilla extract

1 large egg

1 In a blender, combine all the ingredients. Blend for 1 minute, or until well combined.

2 Allow to sit for 5 to 7 minutes for pancake batter and 10 to 12 minutes for waffle batter.

3 Lightly coat a large nonstick skillet or griddle with olive oil spray or coconut oil spray and set over medium heat. Drop batter by ¼ cupfuls onto the hot skillet. Cook for 3 minutes, or until bubbles appear on top and the cakes are golden brown on the bottom. Flip cakes and cook for 2 minutes, or until golden brown on the other side. Repeat with the remaining batter.

4 To serve, top with fresh fruit.

TIP: *Leftover pancakes can be a great healthy snack instead of crackers. Sandwich together with a smear of nut butter and a dab of honey in the middle, and wrap in foil.*

AVOCADO, HONEY, AND CINNAMON SMOOTHIE

—— SERVES 4 ——

At first glance this smoothie sounds strange, but give it a chance and I promise you will be a convert. The creaminess, sweetness, and spiciness blend perfectly together. With this rich drink, a little goes a long way.

2 cups milk alternative of your choice

1 avocado, halved and flesh scooped out

1 cup frozen spinach

1 ripe banana

2 tablespoons honey

1 teaspoon ground cinnamon

In a blender, combine all the ingredients. Blend until smooth.

VANILLA DATE SMOOTHIE

—— SERVES 4 ——

This is another superb way to hide greens in a smoothie! It is sweet and decadent, almost like a dessert—and every ingredient is good for you. Spinach is another option instead of the kale. It will make a room-temperature smoothie.

2 cups milk alternative of your choice

6 pitted dried dates

1 cup frozen kale

¼ cup creamy almond butter

1 tablespoon vanilla extract

In a blender, combine all the ingredients. Blend until smooth.

KALE, BLUEBERRY, MANGO, AND ALMOND BUTTER SMOOTHIE

—— SERVES 4 ——

This is Carmen's favorite smoothie. I rely on it to get her eating those essential vegetables, because even though she's a healthy eater, she is still a toddler, which means we still tussle over green veggies at mealtime. Sharing this is a fun and easy way to sneak them in to her while satisfying my genuine love for all things green and leafy, too! With antioxidant-packed greens and berries, protein, and satiating fats, this smoothie is great after a workout, for breakfast, or to power through a demanding afternoon.

2 cups milk alternative of your choice

1 cup frozen kale

1 cup frozen blueberries

1 cup frozen mango

¼ cup creamy almond butter

In a blender, combine all the ingredients. Blend until smooth.

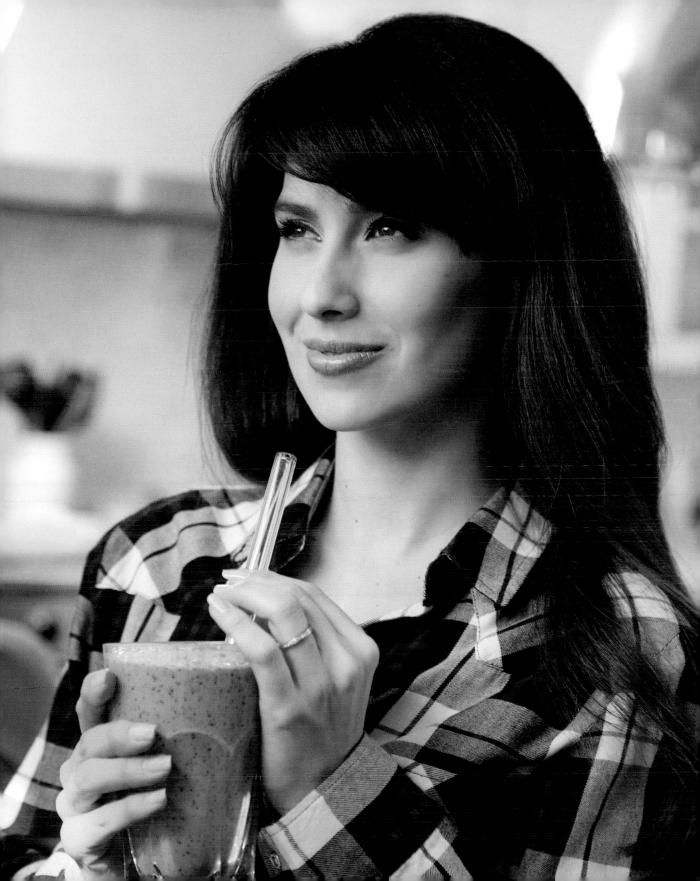

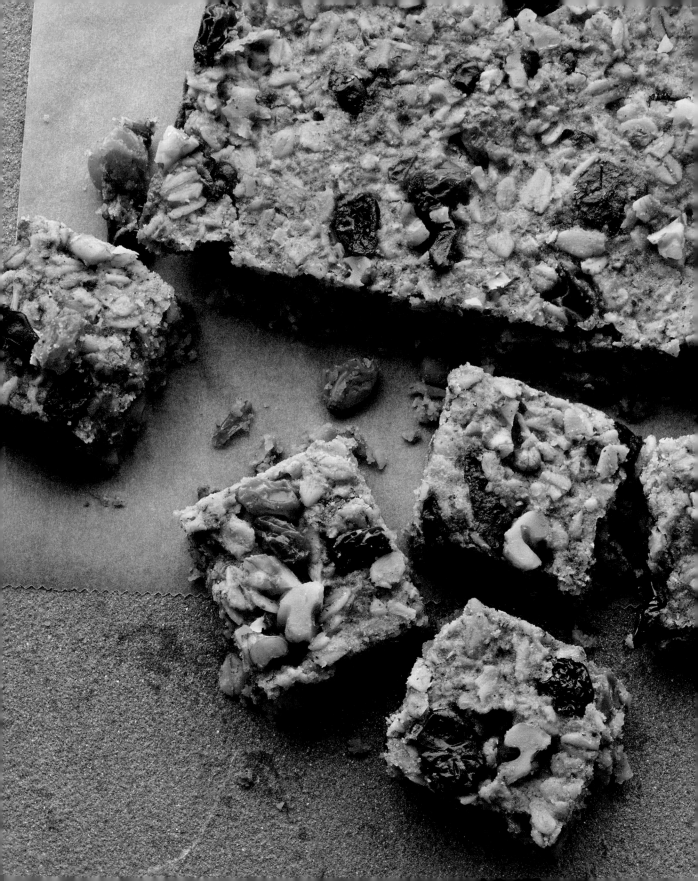

GRANOLA ENERGY BITES

—— MAKES 48 :: SERVING SIZE = 2 PIECES ——

Just because time is short doesn't mean you have to throw good nutrition out the window. These bite-size snacks will satiate hunger on the run. One or two of them will reboot your energy and help you think straight so you can make it through to your next good meal. Don't eat too much of a good thing if you are watching calories. Food is medicine, after all, and it's important to get the right dose.

3 cups rolled oats

1 cup almond flour

2 tablespoons ground chia seeds

⅓ cup golden raisins

⅓ cup dried cranberries

½ cup walnuts, chopped

1 teaspoon ground cinnamon

1 cup almond milk

½ cup applesauce

½ cup olive oil

2 large eggs

1 teaspoon vanilla extract

1 teaspoon grated orange peel

1 Preheat the oven to 350°F. In a 13" × 9" baking dish, overlay a large piece of parchment paper, overlapping all the sides. Coat the paper with coconut oil.

2 In a large bowl, combine the oats, almond flour, chia seeds, raisins, cranberries, walnuts, and cinnamon.

3 In another large bowl, whisk together the almond milk, applesauce, oil, eggs, vanilla, and orange peel.

4 Add the dry ingredients to the wet and stir to combine.

5 Spread the granola mixture onto the parchment paper and push down, making sure the mixture is even and compact. Bake for 25 to 30 minutes, or until browned and dry.

6 Allow to cool completely in the baking dish. Once cool, remove the granola bites by lifting out the parchment paper. Cut into 48 pieces. Store in an airtight container in the refrigerator for up to 1 week.

CORNMEAL-OATMEAL
DARK CHOCOLATE CHIP COOKIES

—— **MAKES 24** ——

My daughter goes crazy for these. They are the ultimate alternative to store-bought cookies! Packed with protein and made with good fats, these cookies are low in sugar but sweet enough to satisfy the itch for a treat.

½ cup melted coconut oil

2 tablespoons crunchy almond butter

½ cup coconut palm sugar

1 teaspoon molasses

4 teaspoons almond milk

1 large egg

1 teaspoon vanilla extract

1½ cups fine yellow cornmeal

½ cup old-fashioned oats

½ teaspoon baking powder

1 cup dark chocolate chips

1 teaspoon sea salt

1 Preheat the oven to 350°F. Line 2 baking sheets with parchment paper or silicone baking mats.

2 In a large bowl, combine the oil, almond butter, sugar, and molasses. With an electric mixer on medium speed, blend for 2 to 3 minutes, or until creamed and fluffy.

3 Add the almond milk, egg, and vanilla and mix on medium speed for 1 minute, or until incorporated.

4 In a medium bowl, combine the cornmeal, oats, and baking powder. Add to the wet ingredients and mix on medium speed for 1 minute, or until incorporated.

5 Stir in the chocolate chips.

6 Scoop 1 tablespoon of the batter, roll into a ball, and place on one of the baking sheets. Repeat with the remaining dough, spacing the balls about 1½" apart. Once complete, sprinkle with the salt.

7 Bake for 13 to 16 minutes, or until lightly browned and set.

8 Cool for 5 minutes on the baking sheets. Transfer to a rack and cool completely, about 30 minutes. Store in an airtight container for up to 1 week (if they last that long!).

CARROT CAKE WITH COCONUT CREAM FROSTING

This luscious dessert epitomizes my philosophy that if you use great ingredients that deliver nutrition to your body—and make it yourself so that you know exactly what's in it—you can enjoy a treat from time to time and drop the guilt. The coconut-milk "frosting" is a revelation—almost sugar-free and rich in good fats that fuel the body and contribute to shiny hair and energized skin. This cake makes 20 small servings; don't go overboard, but do enjoy every bite!

1 cup almond flour plus 2 cups gluten-free all-purpose flour or Healthiest Flour Mix (page 190)

2½ teaspoons ground cinnamon

1½ teaspoons ground ginger

½ teaspoon ground cloves

¼ teaspoon ground nutmeg

2 teaspoons baking soda

1 teaspoon baking powder

1 teaspoon cream of tartar

1 teaspoon salt

¾ cup coconut palm sugar

½ cup olive oil

½ cup applesauce

4 large eggs

3 cups grated carrots

¾ cup unsweetened coconut flakes

1 cup canned crushed pineapple

½ cup milk of your choice (soy, cashew, hemp, almond, dairy)

1 teaspoon plus 1 tablespoon vanilla extract

½ cup golden raisins

½ cup walnuts, chopped (optional)

2 cans (14 ounces each) full-fat coconut milk, refrigerated overnight

1 tablespoon honey

1 Preheat the oven to 350°F. Grease two 8" cake pans and sprinkle with almond flour.

2 In a large bowl, whisk together the flour, cinnamon, ginger, cloves, nutmeg, baking soda, baking powder, cream of tartar, and salt.

3 In another large bowl, whisk together the sugar, oil, applesauce, and eggs. Stir in the carrots, coconut flakes, pineapple, milk of your choice, and 1 teaspoon of the vanilla.

(continued)

4 Add the dry ingredients to the wet and stir until well combined. Add the raisins and walnuts (if desired) and stir until incorporated.

5 Divide the batter between the two prepared cake pans. Bake for 50 to 55 minutes, or until set and golden brown.

6 Allow the cakes to cool for 20 minutes before removing from the pans. Allow to cool completely before frosting.

7 While the cake is baking, make the frosting: Carefully open the cans of coconut milk and pour off the coconut water from each can. Reserve the water for a smoothie or other usage. Spoon out the coconut fat into a blender or Magic Bullet. Add the honey and the remaining 1 tablespoon vanilla and blend for 3 to 5 minutes, or until light and fluffy.

8 Frost the cooled cake with the whipped coconut frosting and serve. Store leftovers in an airtight container in the refrigerator for up to 1 week (if they last that long!).

HEALTHIEST FLOUR MIX

For a little extra effort, you can replace the gluten-free flour (which is essentially processed flour without the gluten) with a super-nutritious alternative. In place of the 2 cups gluten-free flour and 1 cup almond flour, blend together the following:

2 cups almond flour
¾ cup coconut flour

¼ cup tapioca flour
1 teaspoon cream of tartar

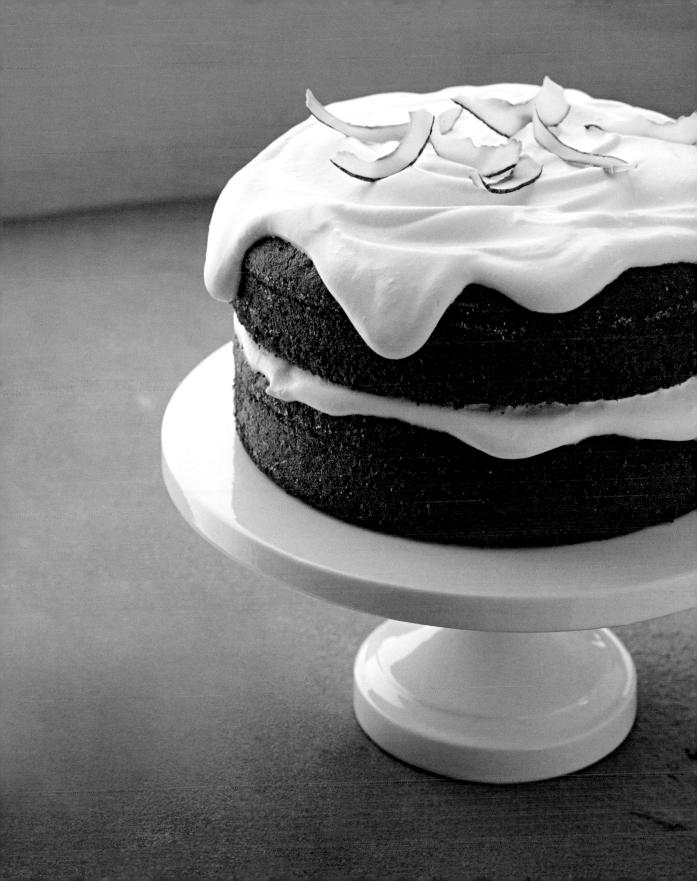

GAZPACHO

—— SERVES 4 TO 6 ——

Gazpacho tastes like summer to me no matter when it's made. Tomatoes picked at the peak of the season are absolutely sublime, and your body loves them because they're bursting with antioxidants! It only takes a couple steps to make this amazing raw soup; it's tomato salad on your spoon and low in calories, too.

4 large tomatoes

½ red, yellow, or orange bell pepper, chopped (about ½ cup)

1–2 cloves garlic

½ cup chopped white onion

⅓ cup peeled and chopped cucumber

¼ cup white wine vinegar

⅛ cup extra virgin olive oil

½ teaspoon salt

½ teaspoon ground black pepper

1 Over a bowl or blender, peel the tomatoes, making sure to save all the juice. In a blender, combine the peeled tomatoes and their juice and the remaining ingredients. Blend until smooth and frothy.

2 Store in the refrigerator for 2 to 3 hours prior to serving. This allows for the flavors to meld and come together. Serve chilled.

TIP: *If you love garlic, let this soup sit in the refrigerator to bring out the garlic flavor, and then reblend and serve chilled.*

ROASTED WHITE WINTER SOUP

—— SERVES 8 ——

This creamy soup is nurturing, warming, and grounding—perfect for chilly days when you want to hunker down and get cozy. White vegetables, often overlooked, are rich in nutrients that boost the immune system, making this winter soup not only a great seasonal staple but also a cold-fighting medicinal brew.

¼ cup olive oil, divided

1 bulb fennel, roughly sliced (about 2½ cups)

1 small cauliflower, roughly chopped (about 3 cups)

4 parsnips, roughly chopped (about 5 cups)

1 large onion, roughly chopped (about 2 cups)

4–6 cloves garlic

1 container (32 ounces) vegetable broth

1 cup dry white wine*

2 cups almond milk

¼ cup apple cider vinegar

1 teaspoon salt

½ teaspoon ground black pepper

1 Preheat the oven to 450°F. Line a baking sheet with parchment paper.

2 Drizzle half of the oil on the prepared baking sheet. Add the fennel, cauliflower, parsnips, onion, and garlic. Drizzle with the remaining oil.

3 Roast for 35 to 40 minutes, or until the mixture is browned, crispy, and tender.

4 During the last 10 minutes of baking time, in a large stockpot or Dutch oven over high heat, bring the broth and wine to a boil. Add the roasted vegetables. Reduce the heat to medium-low and simmer for 15 minutes. Remove from the heat.

5 Using an immersion blender or a tabletop blender, puree until smooth. Add the almond milk, vinegar, salt, and pepper and blend until well incorporated.

6 Return the pureed soup to the pot and bring back to a simmer over medium-low heat (do not boil!). Serve hot.

Alternatives include white wine vinegar, lemon juice, white grape juice, or vegetable stock.

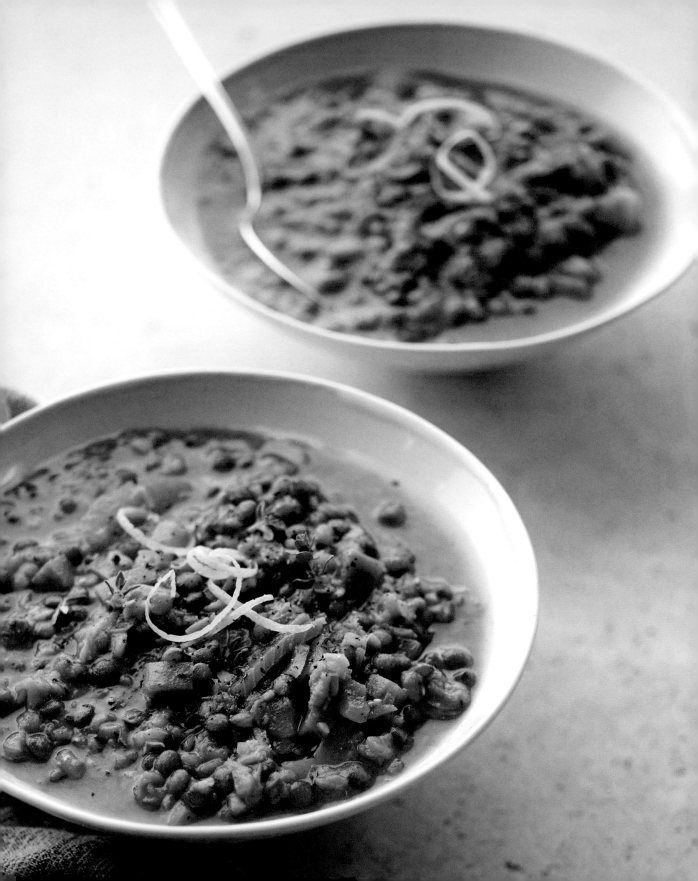

LENTIL SOUP WITH CINNAMON AND LEMON

—— SERVES 10 ——

Great lentil soup is affordable, warming, and so good for you, too. My special twists of cinnamon and lemon have made this one a favorite in my home. If you want to take this up a level, throw in some chopped spinach or kale toward the end of the cooking time. It's so easy to eat your greens when they're served in the same bowl as your soup.

2 tablespoons olive oil

1 sweet onion, diced (about 1½ cups)

1 large carrot, chopped (about 1 cup)

2 ribs celery, chopped (about 1 cup)

4 cloves garlic, minced

2 teaspoons dried thyme

1½ teaspoons ground cinnamon

1 cup dried red lentils

1 cup dried French lentils

1 container (32 ounces) vegetable broth

3 cups water

2 tablespoons grated lemon peel

1 lemon, juiced (about ¼ cup)

1 teaspoon salt

½ teaspoon ground black pepper

1 In a large stockpot or Dutch oven over medium heat, warm the oil. Cook the onion, carrot, and celery, stirring occasionally, for 5 to 7 minutes, or until the vegetables are lightly browned and softened. Add the garlic, thyme, and cinnamon and stir for 30 seconds, or until fragrant.

2 Add the lentils and stir to coat with the spices and oil. Add the broth and water. Increase the heat to high and bring the soup to a boil. Reduce the heat to medium-low, cover, and cook, stirring occasionally, for 45 minutes, or until the lentils are tender and the soup has thickened.

3 Remove from the heat. Add the lemon peel, lemon juice, salt, and pepper and serve.

PASTA PRIMAVERA WITH TOFU

—— SERVES 8 ——

Whether you cook to feed a family or are time-pressed and single, you're probably well versed in making pasta. It can be hard to make it interesting and a challenge to keep it healthy! This is how I pack tons of vegetables into the bowl along with protein from tofu. I prefer whole grain pasta and often use gluten-free brown rice pasta, and the nutritional yeast gives a Parmesan-type flavor. The result is that pasta night goes from lackluster to colorful, tasty, and really fun, too.

1 package (14 ounces) extra-firm tofu

1 package (16 ounces) brown rice pasta or other whole grain pasta

2 tablespoons extra virgin olive oil, divided

6 cloves garlic, chopped

$3/4$ teaspoon salt

$1/2$ teaspoon ground black pepper

1 onion, sliced (about $1/2$ cups)

1 red or yellow bell pepper, sliced (about $1/2$ cups)

2 cups mushrooms, sliced

2 tomatoes, chopped (about 2 cups)

$1/2$ cups dry white wine

1 cup broccoli florets, chopped

1 pound asparagus, trimmed and cut into 2" pieces

$1/4$ cup nutritional yeast

1 tablespoon Dijon mustard

1 Drain the tofu and wrap it in a kitchen towel. Place something like a cast-iron skillet or a cookbook on top of it and allow to sit for 5 minutes. This helps press out some of the excess water. After 5 minutes, unwrap the tofu and cut into 1" cubes.

2 Prepare the pasta according to package directions. Reserve 1 cup of the cooking liquid and then drain the pasta.

3 While the pasta is cooking, make the sauce. In a large, deep nonstick skillet over medium-high heat, warm 1 tablespoon of the oil. Add the tofu and cook, stirring occasionally, for 5 to 7 minutes, or until the tofu is lightly browned and crispy on all sides. Stir in the garlic and season with the salt and black pepper. Transfer the cooked tofu to a small bowl and set aside.

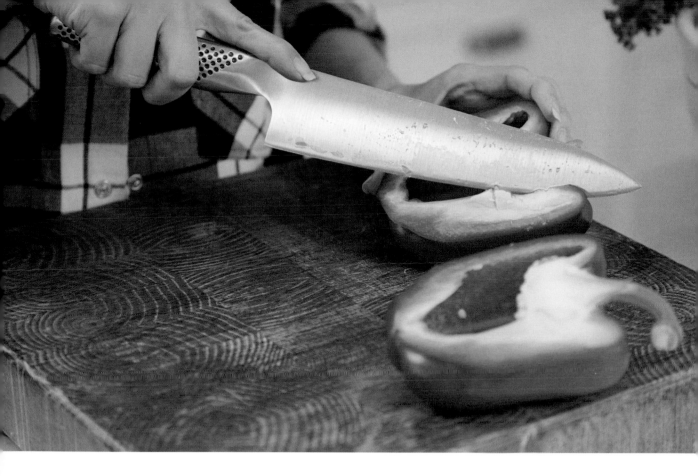

4 In the skillet, add the remaining 1 tablespoon oil, the onion, bell pepper, and mushrooms. Cook, stirring occasionally, for 4 to 6 minutes, or until the vegetables are wilted and starting to caramelize.

5 Add the tomatoes and wine and stir to combine. Cook for 3 to 4 minutes, or until reduced by half.

6 Add the broccoli, asparagus, nutritional yeast, and mustard and stir to combine. Cook for 2 minutes.

7 Stir in the drained pasta and enough pasta cooking liquid to pull the sauce together. Serve immediately.

TIP: *If you're strictly cutting back on carbohydrates, pasta of all kinds is probably off-limits. This recipe works fabulously with roasted spaghetti squash or steamed zucchini noodles made with a spiralizer.*

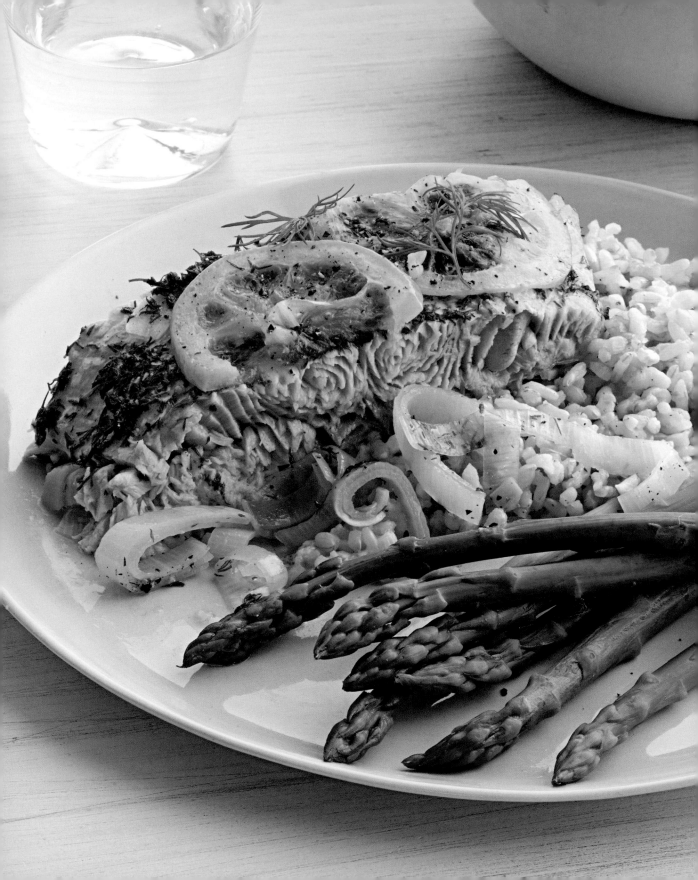

OVEN-ROASTED SALMON WITH HERBS

— SERVES 4 —

This dish makes repeat appearances at my table because it's simple to prepare, delicious, and super easy to clean up. It's great made in the oven or grilled in the summertime, and you don't have to use salmon for it—any firm fish will do. Make extra to use in your lunch bowls or salads. Keeps in the refrigerator for 3 days.

¼ cup extra virgin olive oil, divided

2 large leeks, white part only, sliced (about 1 cup)

1 pound wild-caught salmon

½ cup dry white wine

¼ cup lemon juice

½ teaspoon salt

⅓ teaspoon ground black pepper

4 cloves garlic, crushed

½ cup chopped fresh dill

2 lemons, sliced about ¼" thick

1 Preheat the oven to 350°F. Lay one large piece of parchment paper lengthwise on a baking sheet and then another large piece of parchment paper in the opposite direction.

2 Drizzle 2 tablespoons of the oil onto the bottom of the parchment paper-lined baking sheet. Arrange the leeks on top of the oil. Place the salmon on top and pour the white wine and lemon juice over the salmon. Season with the salt and pepper.

3 Arrange the garlic, dill, and lemon slices on top and drizzle with the remaining 2 tablespoons oil. Close and fold the parchment paper around the salmon, creating a tight packet.

4 Bake for 30 to 40 minutes, or until the fish is opaque.

VEGETABLE AND QUINOA "PAELLA"

—— SERVES 4 ——

Ask a Spanish person about paella and they'll tell you that it takes a lifetime to perfect and a long time to cook! But this simple dinner takes the essence of paella and turns it into a quick, versatile meal. We love it with poached eggs, but feel free to top it with fish, shrimp, chicken, or tofu.

1 tablespoon extra virgin olive oil

1 small onion, diced (about 1 cup)

2 large tomatoes, chopped

4 cloves garlic, minced

1 cup dry white wine

1 tablespoon safflower or saffron

2 cups mushrooms, sliced

1 cup uncooked quinoa

2 cups vegetable broth

1 teaspoon salt

1 teaspoon ground black pepper

3 cups baby spinach

OPTIONAL TOPPINGS
(pick one if using)

4 large eggs

8 ounces cooked chicken

8 ounces cooked shrimp

8 ounces cooked salmon

8 ounces cooked tofu

1   In a large nonstick skillet over medium heat, warm the oil. Cook the onion, tomatoes, and garlic, stirring frequently, for 7 to 10 minutes, or until this "sofrito" is cooked down and the flavors have deepened.

2   While the sofrito is cooking, in a medium bowl, combine the wine and safflower and allow to sit while you continue to cook.

3   In the skillet, add the mushrooms and cook, stirring occasionally, for 3 minutes, or until beginning to brown and caramelize.

4   Add the quinoa and stir to coat with the sofrito. Add the wine mixture and bring to a boil. Reduce the heat to medium-low and cook, stirring occasionally, for 3 minutes.

5   Add the broth, salt, and pepper and stir to combine. Reduce the heat to low, cover, and cook for 15 minutes.

6   Remove the lid, top with the spinach, cover again, and steam for 2 minutes. Stir the spinach into the paella and decide on your topping.

7 For the egg topping, use the back of a spoon to make 4 holes in the paella and drop the eggs into the holes. Cover and cook the eggs for 3 to 4 minutes, or until the whites are set and the yolks are runny. If using one of the other toppings, add to the paella and cook, covered, for the last 3 to 4 minutes to warm through, or if already hot, add on top before serving.

TIP: *Traditional paella has a socarrat, or crust, that forms on the bottom of the pan. This is considered a delicacy among Spaniards and is essential to a good paella. You want this; it is delicious and is made by not stirring the paella during the final cooking time.*

SOFRITO—In Spanish cuisine, sofrito consists of garlic, onion, paprika, and tomatoes cooked in olive oil. It's used as a base.

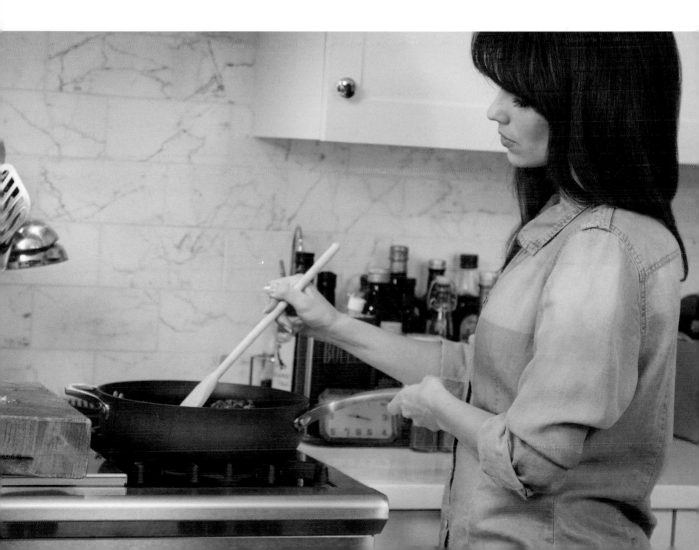

STUFFED PEPPERS

—— SERVES 4 ——

So colorful they'll make you smile when they come out of the oven, stuffed peppers offer yet another way to use your bulk cooked grains. If they're in the fridge, you've already done half the work! The mixture of nutritional yeast and toasted pine nut achieves a cheesy flavor without using dairy. This makes for a simple weeknight dinner and a take-to-work lunch the next day.

¼ cup pine nuts, toasted

½ cup nutritional yeast, divided

4 large yellow, red, or orange bell peppers

2 tablespoons extra virgin olive oil, divided

1 onion, chopped (about 1½ cups)

1 large carrot, chopped (about 1 cup)

1 rib celery, chopped (about 1 cup)

4 cloves garlic, minced

2 cups cooked grains of your choice (quinoa, farro, etc.) or lentils

2 cups tomato sauce

2 tablespoons balsamic vinegar

¼ cup fresh basil, chopped

1 Preheat the oven to 425°F.

2 In a blender or mini chopper, combine the pine nuts and ¼ cup of the nutritional yeast. Pulse until roughly chopped. Set aside.

3 To prepare the peppers, halve each one through the stem and remove the seeds and ribs. Rub the outside with 1 tablespoon of the oil and set in a 13" × 9" baking dish.

4 In a large nonstick skillet over medium heat, warm the remaining 1 tablespoon oil. Cook the onion, carrot, and celery, stirring occasionally, for 5 to 7 minutes, or until softened and lightly golden brown.

5 Add the garlic and stir for 30 seconds, or until fragrant. Add the grains or lentils, tomato sauce, vinegar, basil, and the remaining ¼ cup nutritional yeast and stir to combine.

6 Evenly divide the mixture among the pepper halves. Bake for 40 minutes.

7 Add the reserved topping onto the peppers and bake for 5 minutes.

SHEPHERD'S PIE

— SERVES 8 —

This meat-free version of the traditional comfort food truly hits the spot. Instead of beef or lamb, I combine lentils, mushrooms, and quinoa to achieve a hearty, textured filling. Then, braised greens add iron and calcium, and mashed root vegetables replace the standard mashed potatoes, infusing it with even more vitamin power. This makes a large portion and is even better leftover; use for lunch or freeze half for later.

2 yams, roughly chopped (about 3 cups)

2 large parsnips, roughly chopped (about 2 cups)

3 tablespoons extra virgin olive oil, divided

½–¾ cup milk of your choice (soy, cashew, hemp, almond, dairy)

½ cup nutritional yeast, divided

¾ teaspoon salt

¾ teaspoon ground black pepper

1 onion, diced (about 1½ cups)

1 large carrot, finely chopped (about 1 cup)

2 ribs celery, finely chopped (about 1½ cups)

5 ounces brown button mushrooms, chopped (about 1½ cups)

4 cloves garlic, minced

1 teaspoon dried thyme

1 cup cooked quinoa

1 cup cooked French lentils

2 cups tomato sauce

½ cup frozen peas

Braised Greens (page 168)

1 Preheat the oven to 425°F. Line a baking sheet with parchment paper.

2 In a large bowl, combine the yams, parsnips, and 2 tablespoons of the oil. Spread onto the prepared baking sheet and roast for 25 to 30 minutes, or until tender.

3 In a blender, combine the roasted vegetables, ½ cup of the milk, ¼ cup of the nutritional yeast, salt, and pepper and puree until smooth. Add the extra ¼ cup of milk if needed. Set aside.

(continued)

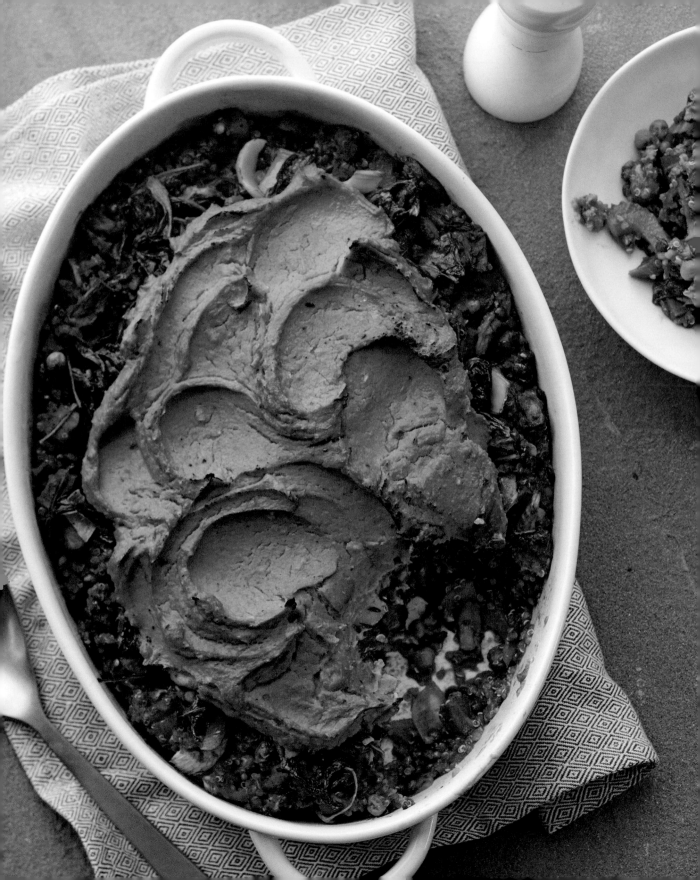

4 In a large skillet over medium heat, warm the remaining 1 tablespoon oil. Cook the onion, carrot, celery, and mushrooms, stirring occasionally, for 7 to 10 minutes, or until softened and lightly golden brown.

5 Add the garlic and thyme and stir for 30 seconds, or until fragrant. Add the quinoa, lentils, tomato sauce, peas, and remaining ¼ cup of the nutritional yeast and stir to combine.

6 To assemble, grease a 2½-quart baking dish with olive oil or coconut oil. Spread the quinoa mixture on the bottom of the baking dish and add the braised greens. Top with the reserved whipped yam mixture and spread evenly. Bake for 15 minutes, or until lightly browned and bubbly.

7 Increase the temperature to broil and, watching the casserole carefully, cook for 2 to 3 minutes, or until lightly browned on top.

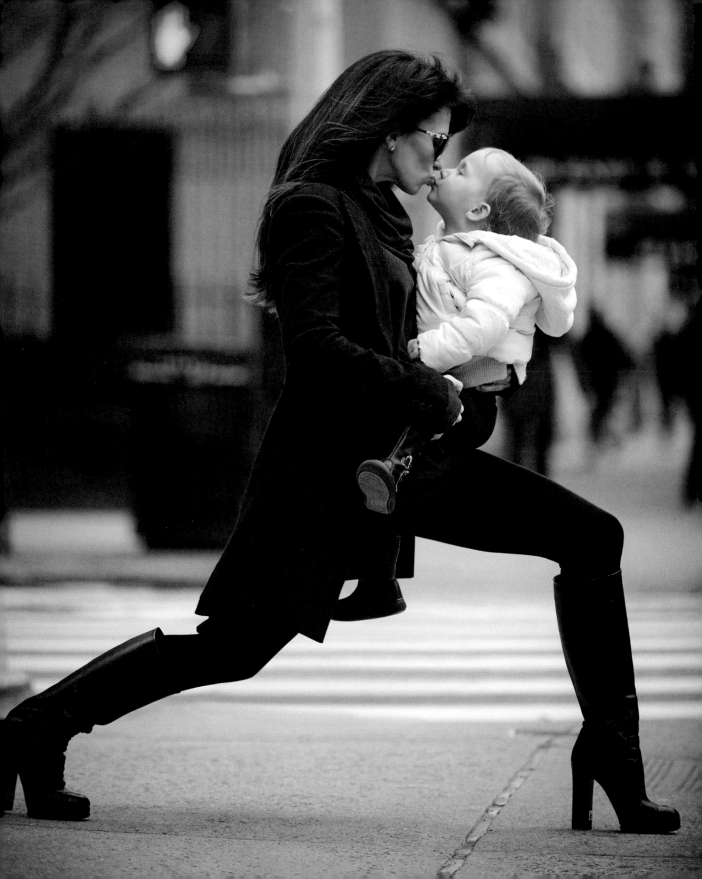

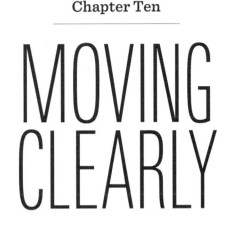

Chapter Ten

MOVING CLEARLY

WHEN IT COMES TO WORKING OUT, MY MANTRA IS "CARPE DIEM." I SEIZE the moment when it appears, no matter how brief it might be, because every little bit counts when it comes to engaging your body. I've always taken a hybrid approach to working out; I believe that movement should be a fully integrated part of your everyday life, not something that you only do working for an hour a day (if you're lucky to get that much time). These days being a mother, fitness has to fit into the pockets and corners of my life (which includes the living room floor, the kitchen counter, or holding on to the back of the high chair). I grab small windows of time to get a run in; take any chance to stretch my body and release tension (Cobra Pose or rolling around with my babies count); and fit daily rounds of ab crunches into stolen moments throughout the day, like getting dressed in the morning or undressed for bed at night. If this makes it sound like I'm always working out, I'm not! I just look through the lens that any place and any time can offer a chance to move. My philosophy is that any amount of movement is time well spent.

And I love it this way, because being in motion is being in my happy place. When I get my husband to go on runs with me, he'll call me his "Annoying Tinker Bell." I zoom about as I work out, running in circles and jumping on curbs, cheering us on. He used to think I was making fun of him; I had to explain I was just happy and having a good time. For me, moving my body has always been my instant way of clearing a dull fog or warding off stormy energy. It literally gets things moving when you're stuck: ideas, hope, and self-belief. It's not that everything in life is better afterward, but a lot of things are. A good workout can change the entire course of the day, inspiring you to choose a healthy meal or get an early night.

I am passionate about lighting the spark to exercise in others because it is more vital today than ever, when the sedentary forces of modern life can literally suck our vitality and well-being away if we let them. "Sitting Is the New Cancer," says one headline. "Sitting Is the New Diabetes," says another. Sitting down all day long—at work, at home, in the car—has become the way of the world, and if we don't actively push against it—with action!—it will tap our bodies and spirits dry.

> I am passionate about lighting the spark to exercise in others because it is more vital today than ever.

The truth is you don't need tons of time working out to stay well and maintain a healthy weight. Science supports this. Long-term statistical studies show that around 30 minutes a day of exercise, with a portion of that being quite vigorous, has significant effects on longevity. Even 15 minutes of vigorous exercise burns a good number of calories while reducing stress, sharpening your thoughts, and helping you sleep. Interestingly, if you dial up your fitness goals—say, you want to significantly change your body shape, gain muscle, or improve performance and beat your own times—then it's mainly about upping intensity, not adding tons more time. Short is always powerful. Done daily, these small fragments do add up.

I don't have a magic wand that always makes working out a cinch. I have my lazy days, and when I've taken a chunk of time off, like after having my children, starting at the bottom again is unpleasant.

But I've got a system that makes everyday exercise enjoyable and tough days manageable. It's built on these simple tenets: Keep it simple, stay consistent, and commit to being present.

THREE IS THE MAGIC NUMBER

I have a general idea of an ideal workout schedule for the week: running most weekdays for a short spell, doing yoga several times a week if I can, and catching a barre class. But I don't count on it happening that way.

My fitness strategy is called the Perfect Three. This brings together three diverse disciplines: cardio, yoga, and toning/sculpting. Together, these are like three legs on a sturdy tripod; they each contribute support for health and well-being, and put together, they create stability. I rely on all three, rotating through them over the course of my week.

Cardio exercise conditions my cardiovascular system, reinvigorates me when I feel tired or dulled, and helps me feel free when life has boxed me in. The endorphins it releases help me to problem solve and think more sharply. Sometimes I get my cardio in through swimming or spin class. But my go-to is running for 30 minutes. I get out on gloomy days and sunny ones, bundling up in the cold and stripping down in the heat.

Yoga gives me flexibility, strength, great circulation and respiration, and balances my mind and spirit. It is not always—in fact, it's not often—a complete, 60-minute class. Any kind of yoga session is an opportunity to give my all—working the length of my body, engaging my mind. This keeps my mind-body connection alive, even on hectic days.

The third leg of the stool is toning and sculpting, which I do through daily exercises that strengthen targeted muscles and sculpt my figure. This makes me feel strong, confident, and fit.

EASY AS 1, 2, 3

1. Cardio burns fat, conditions the metabolism, strengthens the heart, builds stamina, and increases circulation.

2. Yoga promotes mobility, alignment, and strong and elongated muscles and boosts circulation and cardiovascular health while relaxing the nervous system and countering stress.

3. Sculpting and toning fine-tune each muscle, create a chiseled look, and ensure a balanced body.

If you find yourself resisting one of the three disciplines—we've all been there, "I hate to get my heart rate up!" or "Crunches and situps suck!" or "I'm too inflexible for yoga!"—I invite you to let go of old stories and play with something new. If you keep things short and commit to stepping out of your comfort zone, I promise you'll start to discover new capabilities. When done consistently, safely, and at a healthy level of exertion—yes, you do want to sweat!—the Perfect Three really can transform your health and help you attain the figure of your dreams. The truth is you may not like it at the beginning, but eventually you will grow to love it as your body morphs and your endurance increases.

If you can only do one workout, do yoga. For me, it is the epitome of healthy movement: It can get your heart rate up and condition your lungs, target and strengthen specific muscle groups, and stretch and oxygenate your muscles, ligaments, and fasciae. A yoga practice that includes vigorous sessions and slower, strength-focused sequences can be the gateway to an entirely new way of active living.

No matter how you program it, what doesn't change is my golden rule: consistency. Do something. Keep moving. Don't be attached to how much time you have; be attached to how much awareness you can bring to the time you have. Make your workouts deliver bang for the buck.

So don't put off exercise until you have 2 hours to spare to make it to a class in another part of town (then have a shower, blow-dry your hair, and come home). That's great, but it's often out of reach. Instead, make exercise work for your life as you live it daily by creating a sustainable routine—one that fits into the life you already have and adapts to all the interruptions and disruptions that inevitably occur. This is how you make fitness actually *happen*.

Sometimes you have to be super resourceful to pull off exercise when multiple demands are pulling on you. I have a failsafe fashion strategy that really works: black yoga pants! I have a lot of them, and they're practically a daily uniform. When an opportunity opens, I can move comfortably—even if it's doing lunges while the quinoa cooks. Then I throw on boots, a sweater, and a jacket, and nobody in the outside world knows I'm in workout gear. I've even worn this uniform on a night out with stilettos and a cute top—though I've been busted for it by my friends.

Clothes that prime you to move will positively impact your psychology: You'll want to stretch and get up from your desk regularly or do some found-moment exercises (page 238) during the day. You'll be dressed for a workout when the window opens later.

GETTING MORE FROM LESS: THE POWER OF AWARENESS

When yoga taught me to listen to my body, it changed everything about exercising for me. I learned how to take my practice of present-moment awareness off the mat and into a run or more traditional workout, with transforming effects. My runs became more efficient in a shorter amount of time thanks to proper breathing and a focused mind. All my cardio sessions and strengthening exercises became more helpful to my body and less hurtful. I finally tamed the overzealous drive I'd had my whole life, which had contributed to my injury.

When you're tuned out or wrapped up in your thoughts, you almost always end up doing less, quitting earlier, and not integrating the gains you made because you're not even aware of them. Or, worse, you push past messages from your body and get injured. Exercising *with* awareness helps you care for your body wisely and makes any kind of exercise you do effective, at whatever intensity you choose. It makes it more meaningful. You will be amazed by how much your body and mind start to crave physical activity when you're aware and engaged.

Getting there involves putting the Five Living Clearly Principles into motion and having simple workouts that don't take much time. Combine these two things and you will have fitness tools that are easy to use and can be started today!

THE PERFECT THREE MEETS THE LIVING CLEARLY FIVE

Chart 1 Week of Moving Clearly

Think of the Perfect Three as ingredients for a recipe that you customize your way. Review your average week and look for where you already have, or can make, time for exercise. They may be small openings—that's okay! Write down what might work in those windows, depending on your location and responsibilities in that moment. Seeing your average week on a piece of paper or on your calendar can often reveal opportunities you've been missing—like the times you are walking your dog, meeting a friend for coffee, or taking your kid to the park. Get creative: How could you move more in these situations? Where could fitness "fit in" to activities that are otherwise static or slow? And could socializing happen in a new, more physical way? The hard reality is that working out becomes consistent when you prioritize it above other recreational activities. You might also have to consider if there is anything that you could edit.

Your exercise program *will* look different each day. So Wednesday might be about sculpting exercises while cleaning the house and walking to do errands instead of driving, and then on Thursday, a window opens for an hour of yoga. Hurray! It does balance out.

That said, practicing the Five Principles will have you asking, *What do I really need today?* And the answers may differ from what's on your agenda: *I need to run fast and shed the stress of this morning's meetings; I need to roll out a yoga mat and move my joints through a full range of motion and wring out my muscles after hours at a desk; I need to play with my toddler on the floor and laugh and connect together and fire up my energy for the last few hours before bedtime.* This inner guidance can trump your mind's voice that might push you toward repetitive workouts or overly stressful workouts or sabotage your starting at all.

STEP INTO YOUR POWER

You can outsource almost everything in life these days; other people can cook for you, shop for you, organize your closets for you, and walk your dog. But you can't outsource getting fit. Only you can do it, and it requires taking responsibility for yourself. What often gets in the way? Limiting beliefs—those negative thoughts that stop you from starting, even when part of you truly does want to try. Negative beliefs are the voice of the smaller part of you that is clinging to an old-but-comfortable way of being and is scared to change things up. They'll suck your power away if you let them, so if they come up, use my strategies for disarming the four most common limiting beliefs:

1. **I COULD NEVER DO THAT!** Stop comparing yourself to top athletes, trainers, and professionals. Make yourself the star! Your body is as brilliant as any of theirs; you just haven't devoted your life to the same goals they have. Do you really need to be as flexible as a Cirque du Soleil dancer or execute flips like an Olympic gymnast? Probably not. Comparison is a passive act. It keeps you sitting on your butt. Get clear on your own goals, get your sneakers on, and let the fitness models and workout gurus be your teachers, not your idols.

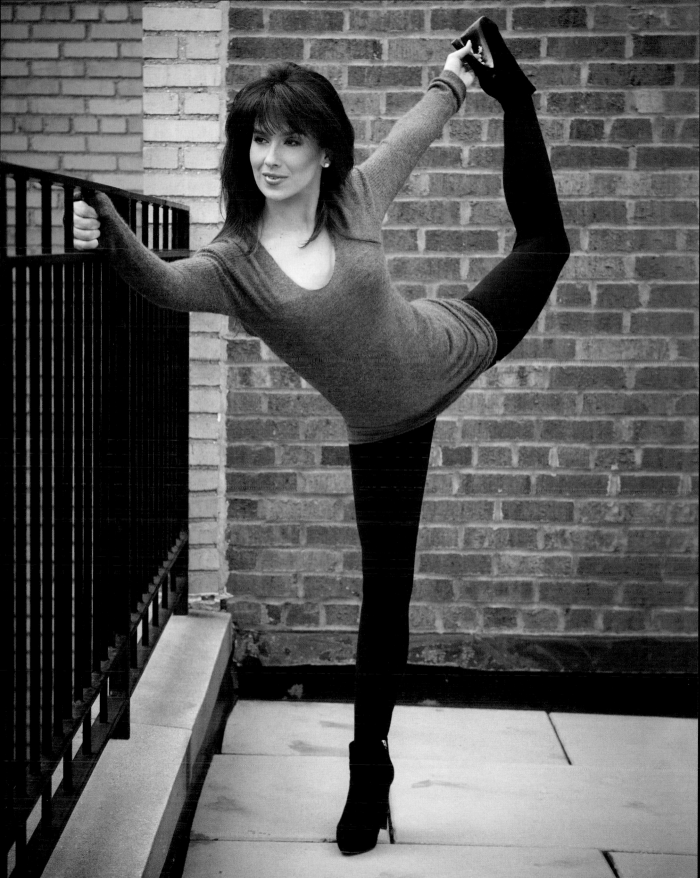

2. **I'LL NEVER HAVE A LEAN/TONED/SHAPELY BODY.** Have you bought into beliefs about your body that are not actually true, like "I'm big boned" or "A bite of ice cream goes straight to my hips"? The human figure is never set in stone. If you eat smartly, exercise regularly with awareness, and get good rest, you *will* see gains and changes. It's unlikely that you are so unique and flawed that these basic laws don't apply to you. Your body is constantly changing—renewing cells, healing imbalances. Change is your very nature. You get to pick the direction this change goes in. There is nothing wrong with you.

3. **I DON'T HAVE TIME TO EXERCISE.** Every person on earth can probably say this. But is it true? Add up the minutes that slipped through your fingers today: 10 minutes hitting snooze, 7 minutes on Facebook, 4 minutes waiting in line at Starbucks, 6 minutes zoning out in the shower, and 3 minutes texting funny pictures to your sister. That's 30 minutes right there. Silly as it sounds, this "personal-time audit" is powerful. Run through your day from waking to sleeping, and count where you've lost minutes to procrastination and distraction. This can all be reclaimed; 10 minutes of yoga can loosen stiff muscles, and 15 minutes of sprints and squats will rev your metabolism when you're sluggish. Turns out you *do* have time!

4. **IF I TRY RUNNING/YOGA/DANCE CLASS, I'LL SUCK AT IT.** There's no reason you should be good at something you've never done before. Take a more playful and relaxed attitude. People who succeed at new things are open-minded and curious—and keep their sense of humor in new situations. They're also kind to themselves and patient. Remind yourself that every day you show up to exercise will see you becoming more capable, fitter, stronger, and leaner. This is about progress, not perfection.

Now that we've got those cleared up, let's move on!

CARDIO

Doing cardio means getting your heart rate up and increasing blood circulation in your body for sustained periods of time. It burns calories and boosts metabolism, helping you to maintain your weight, or lose weight if that's a goal. It conditions and strengthens your heart—vital for health and longevity—and it initiates a cascade of feel-good chemicals that counter stress, depression, and fatigue and help you think more clearly. Moving swiftly is probably the fastest way I know to light the spark of optimism inside; cardio is a power tool for clearing a foggy state and putting possibility within reach.

Though we all know we *should* push ourselves to move quickly and pump the heart, many of us do anything to steer clear of it—and that includes plenty of yoga practitioners! Sweating, pushing hard, possibly getting winded from exertion because you've never really done it—the thought of it can be uncomfortable, if not distressing. And it is true that getting in the saddle with cardio exercise, or getting back on the saddle after a break, is hard. But not for long. By taking it slow and steady, showing up consistently, and staying present while you do it, cardio becomes first manageable and then enjoyable. No matter what shape you're in today, you will see small progressions tomorrow and the day after: running one block farther or two, breathing easier, or biking to a faster pop song than before. By reflecting on what you did (see "Exercise Reflection" on page 226), you'll notice these gains, which grows your self-esteem—the best motivation there is!

CARDIO FOR EVERY BUDGET, SCHEDULE, AND WEATHER CONDITION

- ▶ Power walking and running
- ▶ Stair climbing at home or work
- ▶ Elliptical machines at the gym
- ▶ Boot camp class in the park
- ▶ Jump rope and kettle bells in your backyard

- ▶ Dancing and swimming
- ▶ Rowing, cycling, and cross-country skiing (in nature or on stationary equipment)
- ▶ Jogging with your stroller or trail-hiking with your baby in a carrier

The goal of Living Clearly is to create a habit of doing cardio for 30 minutes three or four times a week. These sessions should get your heart rate elevated and your body working quite hard. When that becomes comfortable, add another day. The pace you keep will depend on your age, current condition, and any physical limitations; if you move at a pace where you can speak in choppy sentences, but not full ones, you're at a healthy moderate zone (50 to 65 percent) of capacity. You can build off this base later, if you like, with more advanced practices that push you harder, like high-intensity workouts. But the challenge of completing 30 minutes of highly active, "moderate" movement every other day is quite enough to start.

Do whatever is the simplest way to lace up your sneakers and go before excuses get in the way. Remember, it's not so much *what* you do but *how* you do it.

Depending on your current fitness level, you might have to keep your pace dialed down at first or alternate between slower and faster phases—that's fine. Just remember the golden rule: Consistency is more important than duration. Short, frequent cardio sessions are less stressful on the body than long, endurance-style sessions and can have greater metabolic impact if they're intense enough, helping you to burn fat throughout the day. So rather than wait until a 90-minute time slot opens for a run or bike ride on the weekend, grab that 25-minute window that opens today and jump into training time.

I'd be lying if I said that starting any routine was easy. Thirty minutes can feel like an agonizing eternity at first! Your mind will yell, "Are you crazy?" and come up with a thousand excuses to stop. Give yourself permission to be bad at it for a while. Just show up, be mediocre, and then show up again. As every other person who ever started working out will attest, gradually it starts getting easier.

TIMING IS EVERYTHING

Find a time of day when you can consistently get active. Early-morning exercisers tend to be more consistent than evening ones because the day doesn't get the best of them. But midday breaks might prove addicting as they refresh and reboot your body and mind. Try different options at first, and jot notes in your calendar about what you did, how it felt, and any pros and cons. This will help you find the windows of time that work best for your life.

For years, I had exercise-induced asthma; my lungs would burn as I ran, and I'd be forced to stop even though I had energy to spare. I always felt like I was gasping for breath (a stressful sensation that unconsciously triggers your fight-or-flight response). Yoga gave me the solution: By applying the steady nose-breathing technique from my yoga mat to running, as well as to most other cardio exercises, I began to condition and strengthen my lungs tremendously. It was awkward at first. Inhaling and exhaling only through my nose, I could only get a short way. I'd have to stop, catch my breath, and then start again. I was stopping all the time! But the burning sensation and asthmatic episodes began to diminish. The more I practiced this Runner's Breath (see page 219), the more my lung strength grew, and I ran longer distances without pausing. The lungs get stronger, just like any other muscle. Today, I can run for miles inhaling and exhaling through my nose exclusively; I feel calm and easy, not stressed.

Running and Walking—The Ultimate Easy, Adaptable Cardio Exercise

When you get in your stride with running, it can make you feel like a kid again—jumping for joy and bursting with energy. It's always been my go-to, but I had to learn to run wisely as running improperly definitely contributed to my hip fracture. Today, I approach it with moderation, using my Five Principles to listen to my body and keep my tendency to overtrain in check. No amount of calories burned is worth the suffering I experienced.

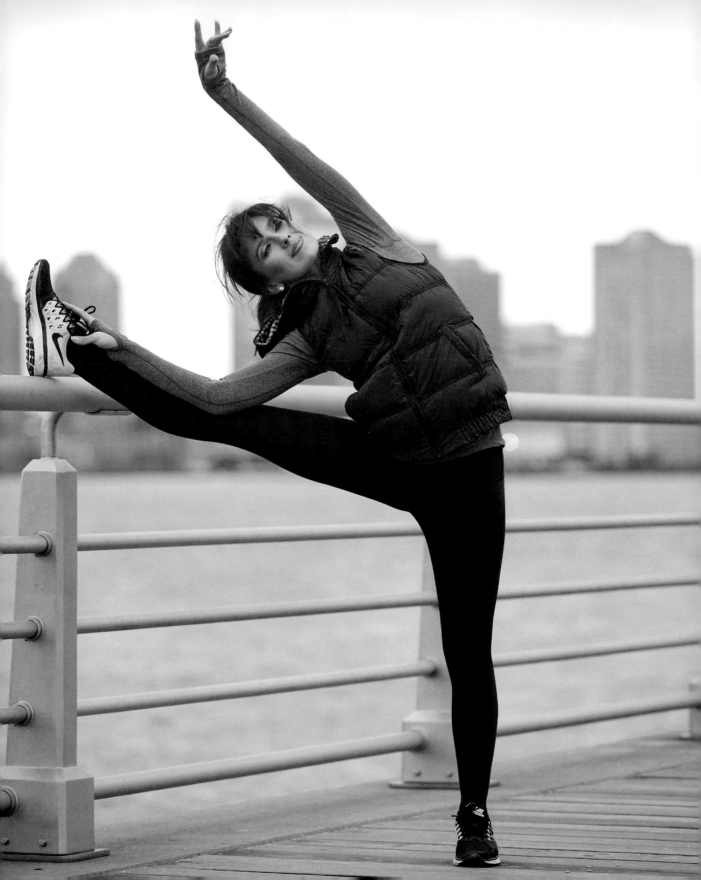

Power walking, running's slower sibling, is a tremendous alternative, especially if you struggle with running but want to target the same muscle groups. It is low impact, which helps if you have injuries or feel that gentler is better for you. If done at a good pace, power walking can really get your heart pumping, and it can even work your butt and hamstrings more than running.

I recommend having these simple cardio exercises in your rotation, because no matter where you are in the world or how much time you have, running and power walking will adapt to your limitations and schedule.

SEVEN TIPS FOR RUNNING CLEARLY

1. **ADJUST YOUR FORM.** Engage your core by bringing your belly button toward your spine while slightly tilting your body weight forward. Relax your shoulders and let your arms move naturally at your sides; keep your hands soft. Scan your body for tension as you run and let go of it.

2. **USE RUNNER'S BREATH.** Breathing is *everything* in running. On your next fast walk or run, try to inhale and exhale only through your nose, or exhale through your mouth as your intensity increases. Stop and reset every time you lose this breath. The better your lungs work, the more efficient your cardio session will be and the more clear-minded you will feel as you move.

3. **KEEP MOVING.** Your goal is to keep your heart rate up. The only time to stop is if you are taking a break to retrain your breath or if you need to take care of your body. At traffic lights, jog in place or find another way to keep your heart rate up. Notice your mind coming up with reasons to stop; ask yourself if you can let that go.

4. **LIVE THE PROCESS.** Be patient with the process of getting in shape. Trust that slow and steady wins the race. When I broke my hip and started running from square one again, it was a big knock to my ego, but guess what I learned? Ego has nothing to do with working out. It was ego that led me to break my hip in the first place. Trust that your body is brilliant and that if you go slow and steady, you will gradually run farther. Never be embarrassed; you are on track to change.

5. **KEEP IT FRESH.** Figure out what kind of runner you are. I am a big fan of outdoor running because I love to see the scenery and change up my course. My body feels much better outside than on a treadmill. In the city, I use music to fire me up and give me much-needed "me" time. In nature or on the beach, I run in silence. Running with a buddy is fun because it makes the time go by quickly, but running alone is therapeutic, a time to be alone with your thoughts, your breath, and the Five Principles. Change it up from time to time to keep yourself engaged.

6. **CREATE A ROUTINE.** It's better to do three shorter runs in the week than one very long run. My personal rule is 30 minutes at a time—with occasional 45-minute runs if I'm having a great time. I never go over that. That makes a run easier to schedule and protects your body.

7. **DRESS FOR SUCCESS.** A favorite ensemble that makes you feel jazzed and sporty really puts a pep in your step! It's purely psychological, but if your running uniform makes you feel like a superhero, you're more likely to run like one. I wear my signature black leggings, a puffy vest over a running bra, and my gigantic headphones (you can't miss me when I'm wearing them). If it's cold, I wear a long-sleeved workout top under the vest (the key here is to keep my core warm). In the summer, I wear a light vest and nix the shirt underneath. It's my personal running ritual: Getting all suited up gets my body and mind ready to fly.

10:10:10

A fun way to work with the Perfect Three is to combine them all in one workout, with 10 minutes of cardio, 10 minutes of yoga, and 10 minutes of toning work. You'll blast through 30 minutes because your mind is anticipating the change to come. You can also do this over the course of one day, finding three pockets of time, one in the morning, one in the afternoon, and one in the evening.

Yoga for Running and Walking

A simple way to enhance your running or walking is to start with yogic postures that warm up the legs, loosen the hips, and stretch the front and back body. They also help you become present to what you are about to do. The ab workout done afterward is extra effective because of the heat you just created inside; dig deep and let the fire in your core power you through. Pigeon Pose offers a moment of reflection to integrate your work and treat your hips to a deep stretch.

BEFORE
LOW LUNGE

From your hands and knees, step your right foot forward. Lift your chest and place both hands on your right quad above your knee. Push your hips forward while pointing your back toes, slightly arching to open your chest. Feel the stretch in your left hip flexor. Take five breaths, and then switch sides.

STANDING HALF HERO'S POSE

From a standing position, holding on to a chair or wall, slightly soften your right knee (your standing leg). Bend your left knee completely and reach around to grab your left foot with your left hand, pulling the heel inward toward your buttocks. Shift your left knee down and back so that they line up with your right to maximize the hip flexor stretch while stretching your quads. Take five breaths, and then switch sides.

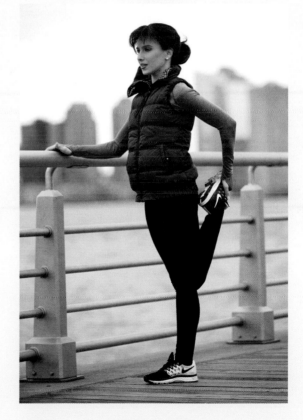

AFTER
HILARIA'S CORE WORKOUT *(page 236)*

PIGEON POSE *(page 115)*

THE FIVE IN MOTION

Any kind of exercise can be a canvas for practicing staying present. In a challenging workout, you are pushing and puffing so hard that all thoughts of the outer world stop. In that moment, the sensations inside are so strong, your mind is transfixed by what's happening. All it can think is, "Holy cow!" And when you fall on the floor at the end, the heightened awareness of every sensation—breath, sweat, release—ensures your mind is not ticking through to-do lists or mundane thoughts. You feel fully alive and fully present.

This has a positive side effect—a greater respect for your own body. The more awareness you have of the better state you just created, the more awe you will feel for your physical form—and the less frustration you will have with its perceived limitations or imperfections. You will notice that it is, frankly, an extraordinarily designed machine.

Using the Five Principles in all my workouts has helped me get to know myself so much better; they're now as indispensible as my Nike sneakers or my puffy running vest. Today, they help me stay present, clearer on what I want and need, and they help me let go of any struggle. They are the best type of workout gear you can have for free!

❶ Perspective

QUESTIONS: *How will I feel after I exercise? How will I feel if I don't?*

Whether you are an experienced athlete or newly active, activating perspective will help you pull your sneakers out of the closet on tough days and keep going when you might otherwise give up. Remind yourself how accomplished and energized you feel after you move. Recall a moment when you've felt the burning of intensity followed by the euphoria of release, like during the Activation and Release exercise on page 40. Then summon up a vision of the "you" that exercise is helping to create. *I am becoming: fit, agile, lean, sexy, strong, healthy for my kids, as fast as my partner, stunning in my wedding dress.* These are your big-picture goals.

Any time you get blocked by negative thoughts and limiting beliefs, apply the six-step Perspective Process.

1. Pause and catch that negative thought before it gains traction.

2. Zoom out to see the macro view. Remember, you have goals and aspirations that are bigger than this small moment.

3. Ask the questions: *How will I feel when I complete the run/bike ride/yoga session? How will I feel if I don't?*

4. Buoyed by that awareness, make a positive choice.

5. In the grand scheme of things, how much time is this really going to take?

6. Burning sensations are temporary.

The exciting news is that activating perspective becomes easier the more you exercise. Each time you experience good sensations in your body, you are making positive associations, which can override any resistance that stands in your way.

❷ Breathing

QUESTIONS: *Am I aware of my breath? Can I make it fuller, steadier, and more intentional?*

One of the reasons people hate to work out (particularly cardio) is because they don't know how to breathe properly and do not have sufficient strength in their lungs. That burning sensation in your chest totally sucks, right? I promise: Any exercise you do is transformed by conscious breathing. Each time you prepare to work out, take a moment to establish a good breathing pattern of steady breath through the nose. This will start generating heat, loosening tension, and creating more space. Keep any music off right now. Instead, let your breath be the soundtrack to your movement.

Start with the Mountain Pose breathing exercise from page 66, breathing in and out of your nose for 1 to 2 minutes. Then link your inhales and exhales to your stretching as you increase circulation, wake up your lungs, and soften tense spots. Sweep your arms overhead and move into Forward Fold, elevate into a tiptoe Relevé, and then step sideways into a Wide Squat. Get creative and play here; the point is to move freely, choosing your reverse positive.

Let your breath be the driver for each movement and use this warmup to truly get *in* to your body. It might look like this: Inhale, do a big stretch; exhale, fold into a bend. Inhale, draw your attention into your body; exhale, drop into your body. Inhale, visualize your lungs getting conditioned; exhale, let them wring out tension and stress. Repeat five times.

Use the Runner's Breath on page 219 during low- and moderate-intensity exercise. As intensity increases, keep the nasal inhale, but exhale through the mouth if you need. Steady nose breaths may be challenging at first, but they get easier with practice. This small-seeming detail feeds big gains in quality of life because the more efficient you become at supplying your body and brain with oxygen, the more clearly you think and feel.

❸ Grounding

QUESTIONS: *Can I feel my entire body? Do I feel fully here? Can I feel my weight sinking into the ground?*

Mindless exercising might get you through a workout, but it creates a missed opportunity for recruiting more of your energy and willpower (and it creates a potential liability; you can miss all kinds of important cues from muscles, tendons, and ligaments).

Try turning off distractions, putting down the phone, and grounding into the earth before you begin working out. The style of yoga I teach emphasizes sinking or rooting the body into the substance of the earth, whether it's through the feet, back of the body, front of the body, or hands—whatever body part is connected to the ground in that moment. It is about really feeling the substance of your body. Remember, there is no reason to shy away from feeling the weight and density of your body. You are created out of substance after all (if you weren't, you'd be invisible!). Grounding is about feeling *you* and creating a state of presence where you are content to inhabit your body. That's why I love starting a cardio workout or even just a restorative walk with a few yoga poses. They help bring you firmly into the physical body so you feel more sensations and get more out of the workout that follows. It's also about feeling what you have to work with. Namely, you!

Try this: Do the grounding exercise on page 79 as your warmup. Then take it into your first steps on a fast walk or run. Push the weight of your substance off the substance of the earth with each stride if you're walking or running. Throughout your workout, you can return to the grounding exercise several times: Pause, flex your feet, and relax them, and then shift your weight from foot to foot again. You will be amazed how this brings you back from distraction and helps access more energy and strength. (You can also do this while swimming. "Grounding" in the water means consciously engaging each pull of your arm or kick of your leg through the substance of the water, pressing against it and pushing off it.)

These grounding experiences help you work your muscles more intentionally, transforming not just the way you look but the way you feel about yourself. Instead of wishing you were lighter or shaped differently, you may find you feel more accepting of your frame and more grateful for your body's abilities. Making peace with yourself is your greatest source of strength.

❹ Balance

QUESTIONS: *Can I find my fire and passion to feel amazing? Should I dial it up and work harder? Should I dial it down and rest and recover?*

Balance in exercise can be literal, like holding Tree Pose on one graceful leg, as well as mental: *Am I working my body hard enough or too hard?* You achieve both kinds of balance when you connect to your core. An easy way to do this is to include the core workout sequence (page 236) after any cardio you perform. Additionally, practice engaging the core while running, biking, or moving quickly through yoga poses to help you move efficiently without injury.

You also have a mental-emotional core. It's your center, the seat of your will. This core is the place where the fire of your passion lives; it's also where your wisdom tells you if you're taking the right action for your current needs. So it is equally essential to engage on the path to fitness. As you're exercising, ask yourself, *Do I need to push and sweat harder and get through this discomfort to get juiced about my life? Can I "fire myself up" more, get more excited, and feel more passion? What greater goal am I moving toward?* Use that goal to feed the flames. *What do I need both physically and emotionally?*

Stoke Your Fire

To determine if you are in your fitness sweet spot, notice if you are able to carry on a breezy conversation as you work out. If yes, you're not working vigorously. Try to push a little harder. If you can barely get a word or two out, you are working at your max. This is great for a sprint or fast interval; just follow with a few moments of strolling recovery before you do it again. The "choppy-sentence" trick keeps you at a moderate zone. If you tend to stay in the strolling zone, apply a shot of perspective when you push a little harder: Tell yourself that this burn is temporary and you will feel triumphant after you're done. One of the best ways to get comfortable with being a little uncomfortable is to take group classes where the whole room is focused on making it through. Experience it enough times and you'll be able to take that same vigor to solo workouts.

If you practice being honest (and probably 75 percent of people will typically need to push a bit harder than back off) and learn to rev it up on some days while resting and restoring on others, you can truly develop responsibility and self-reliance in your exercise program, which is something no trainer or gym membership can give you.

❺ Letting Go

QUESTIONS: *Am I holding on to tension? Am I taking this too seriously? Could I let it go and have fun?*

Sure, there are lots of serious reasons we exercise, but it's also to let go of tension, loosen our grip on life, and play again. So whether you're off for a run or a weights session or a yoga class, check your ego at the door. Your ego might care about doing things right, keeping up with other people, or bettering them, but your innocent childlike self wants to express itself through movement. It wants to dance at the stoplights and leap over puddles and make silly faces and get it all wrong and wave at strangers.

How can you let loose a little and honor that child inside? Before you start your workout—be it cardio *or* yoga—jump in place, shake, and twist from side to side. Let go of what happened today, let go of what you have to do later. Upbeat music can be your friend

---

Exercise Reflection

After you're done with your workout, lie down for a few moments (this might mean on the mat in the gym; it's okay to do that!) or take a moment to stand still and tune in. Feel your heart beating, your muscles burning and then relaxing, your emotions soaring and then quieting, the rush of accomplishment. Notice how your calm postexercise body creates a calm mind.

This moment of reflection is when all the hard work integrates and becomes part of you. It gets seared into your muscle memory (helping you next time you run through the Perspective Process) and makes exercise part of who you are. Little by little, this is how you get shaped into someone who loves to move.

And please give yourself a high five. You just worked your brilliant body. It might have been simple according to other peoples' standards, but who cares? You did it!

Putting the Five Principles in Motion

When I'm struggling to motivate myself to work out, I play what I call the Activation Game. I say to myself, *Okay, mind, help me train the body today.* The mind loves to be important, so I give it a job to do instead of letting it sabotage things. I will run through the Five Principles before I work out and return to them during the workout to stay present, connect into the experience—and not quit early! Once I've got the first few workouts under my belt, I start feeling back on track; I remember that in a few weeks I'll be back to my normal fitness level. And it becomes fun again.

Before your next workout, take 1 minute to run through all of the Five Principles in order. This is quick, but it can powerfully commit you to the effort ahead.

1. Connect to your long-term goals.

2. Breathe consciously to draw your mind inward and warm up the body.

3. Root down into the body to get grounded, turn away from distraction, and get into the present.

4. Find the fire and the guidance at your core.

5. Then let go of expectations, shake out tension, smile, and get started!

here. After all, how often do you get to dance and party? This might be your only chance of the day.

During your workout, don't care quite so much about outcomes and achievements; just be in the experience without judging or overthinking. In yoga, once one posture is completed, you cannot get it back; you must let it go and move forward. Applying that awareness to every exercise session is liberating.

And notice if you can release tension from parts of your body that don't need to be working, like your shoulders, fists, or brow. Only work as hard as you need to. Be smart and efficient with your energy. You do not need to burn calories in your eyebrows by crunching them in a frown! You should be a well-oiled machine, using every part efficiently and effectively.

Yoga for Biking

The first time I went to SoulCycle, one of New York City's legendary spin classes, I was shocked at how hard it was. The only reason I made it to the end was that I wanted to retain some dignity! By developing good form, I learned to love it and created a yoga class especially for SoulCycle devotees called Soul Yoga. Yoga and spinning go well together because flexibility and a greater range of movement help you to get more out of the workout. The following postures strengthen and stretch muscles that typically get overworked and support you to ride well, whether you're on a road bike, on a stationary bike, or sweating wildly in spin class.

BEFORE
LOW LUNGE VARIATION TO CHIN TO SHIN

From your hands and knees, step your right foot forward, lift your chest, and place both hands on your right quad just above your knee. Bring your left hand to the floor and bend your left knee, lifting your left heel toward your buttocks. Twist your body to the right, grabbing your foot with your right hand. Now, rotate your right shoulder forward so that both shoulders are attempting to face forward, pressing your pelvis downward to stretch the psoas and quad. Take five breaths, and then switch sides.

Frame the front foot with your hands, curling your back toes under, popping the left knee off the mat, and straightening both legs. Bring the back foot in a couple of inches (up to 12 inches) so both feet are grounded on the floor with the back toes slightly turned out. Inhale flex your foot (optional), half lift your body, pulling up through your core; twist your sternum slightly toward your front knee and exhale fold forward over your leg. Take five breaths, and then switch sides.

AFTER
DOWNWARD FACING DOG
Peddling Feet Out *(page 46)*

SEATED SPINAL TWIST
(page 125)

SEATED FIGURE FOUR
From Seated Spinal Twist, extend your left leg straight and butterfly open your right knee, ankle resting on your left quad just above your knee, sole of your foot facing the left wall. Flexing your right foot to protect the knee joint, fold forward over your left leg. Take five breaths, and then switch sides.

BETTER BIKING TIPS

Use your core: Pull your belly button toward your spine so your center is engaged, your shoulders are soft, and your arms are extended long. Breathe into the tightness.

Also try using the Runner's Breath, page 219, and inhale only through your nose. Focus on exhaling the burn out of your lungs and out of your muscles, and know that your lungs will get stronger!

Yoga for Swimming

Swimming is an incredible low-impact workout that challenges the breath and gives wonderful tone to the body. When I started swimming, I was fresh out of my wheelchair and even doing five laps with a paddleboard was exhausting. Little by little, I graduated to a breaststroke kick. Then I tried without the board. I did just one length and thought I was going to sink! But I stuck with it, and every day I made it one more length, until gradually my lungs and body stopped burning with effort as I worked. What I discovered was a heart-pumping, exhilarating workout that left me vibrant and full of life after each swim and then happily exhausted at night, getting terrific sleep.

BEFORE
SEQUENCE: PUPPY POSE, DOLPHIN PLANK, EAGLE POSE, HILARIA TUCK AND CURL

1. **PUPPY POSE.** Starting on your hands and knees, walk your hands out in front of you, keeping your elbows straight. Your hips should be over your knees and your toes pointed. Lower your chest toward the ground with an arch in your back, until your forehead meets the floor or a folded towel. Extend your arms as actively and as much as possible, and press your hands into the ground, spreading your fingers, while pulling your hips back. To move more deeply into the pose, place your chin to the floor and look forward. Take five breaths.

2. **DOLPHIN PLANK.** Shift your weight forward, place your hands, forearms, and elbows firmly into the floor, and walk your feet back into Dolphin Plank/Forearm Plank. Hold to work your core and pelvic floor, strengthen your quads, and tone the deltoids (important muscles for swimming). Take 10 breaths.

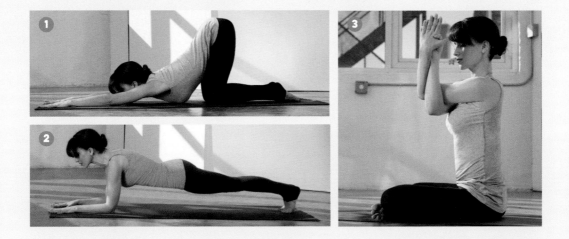

THE LIVING CLEARLY METHOD

3. **EAGLE POSE.** Push back to sit, kneeling on your heels (sitting on a chair or standing is fine, too). With your hands reaching above your head, palms facing inward, wrap your arms around each other, right arm under your left, crossing your upper arms. Keeping your arms as high as possible, continue to work your right arm around your left in a counter-clockwise motion, creating another cross in your arms just below your wrists. Attempt to press your palms together in a twisted prayer. (*Alternate:* Grab opposite shoulders, or elbows, if pressing your palms together is too challenging.) Bring your elbows up toward your nose, out away from you, and then down toward the floor as your shoulder blades stretch apart from your thoracic spine. Take five breaths. Unwrap your arms, and give yourself a shoulder roll. Switch sides.

4. **HILARIA TUCK AND CURL.** With your fingers interlaced behind your head, exhale tuck your chin and round your cervical and thoracic spine, looking down at your belly button, bringing your elbows together. Inhale open your elbows wide, move your chin up and away, arch your upper spine, and look at the ceiling. Do this five times.

AFTER
WIDE STRADDLE, HAPPY BABY, APANASANA

1. **WIDE STRADDLE.** Sitting on a folded towel if necessary, straddle your legs wide enough to feel your inner thighs opening and stretching from your groin. Flexing your feet with your knees pointing upward, walk your hands forward, lowering your torso toward the floor. Take five breaths. Roll back up, place your right forearm on the floor in front of your right leg, sweep your left arm up and over your head, and stretch your body to the right, feeling the opening on the left side deeply between the intercostal muscles. Take five breaths, and then switch sides. Close your legs slowly.

2. **HAPPY BABY.** Lie down and bring your feet up and straddle your knees wider than your belly. Support your head with a towel or pillow if needed. Holding the outsides of your feet (or ankles, shins, or hamstrings), continue to open your knees wider than your torso, gently aiming your knees toward the floor up by your armpits, pulling down with your hands. Rock from side to side, opening one and then the other. Take five breaths.

3. **APANASANA.** Drawing your knees tightly into your chest, reach your arms around your knees and embrace yourself. Grab opposite wrists, forearms, or elbows. Keep your head on the floor or a towel and feel your lower back and hip flexors stretch. Take five breaths.

BETTER SWIMMING TIPS
To help use your leg muscles to the max, engage your core and extend through your legs. Press the water away with each stroke—grounding in liquid—to increase effort and hone lean muscles. And lather your hair with conditioner before you swim to protect it from the chlorine or salt!

BEFORE

A good teacher should warm you up well once class begins. The only ground rules are to avoid eating a major meal 2 to 3 hours before yoga class, if you can, and to be well hydrated.

If you're new, get to class a little early so you can pick a good spot. Don't hide at the very back or squeeze against the side wall. Put yourself smack in the middle of the room so that you can see others no matter which way you face. They can guide you when you need visual cues.

Don't be nervous: Yoga is playtime! Be curious and have fun. And remember: you are the expert on you; only you can monitor how you are feeling in the class. You can rest in Child's Pose at any point. This is called taking responsibility for your own practice.

AFTER

Take a moment to notice the awareness you just created inside. Try to hold on to as much of it as you can; don't just give it all away and get caught back up in the world's demands within 20 seconds! Move quietly and slowly as you leave your class. This will help you take your newly found calm and clarity off the mat.

THE YOGA SEQUENCES

The five sequences in Part One of this book are designed to give you building blocks that you can play with in various ways as part of your fitness program. Use them individually—each one lasts roughly 10 minutes—or put them together, doing two or even three in a row. Turn them into a skyscraper of a workout by doing cardio before, a challenging ab-strengthening sequence during, and a longer resting pose at the end.

Each sequence is designed as a gateway to one of the Five Principles. You might gravitate toward the one that suits how you are feeling that day or the state you need to be in. Of course, each one offers the opportunity to practice all five. Yoga practice is what the Five Principles were born from; when done with intention, every yoga sequence you do allows for the dawning of perspective, the deepening of breath, the grounding into the earth, the connecting to the center, and a releasing letting go.

USING THE FIVE YOGA SEQUENCES

There are lots of ways to use the yoga sequences in this book to complete the yoga portion of the Perfect Three. Here are some options.

► Do one of them when you have a 10- to 15-minute window. End with 1 minute of Savasana.

► Repeat the same flow for a 20- to 30-minute practice. End with 3 minutes or more of Savasana.

► Mix and match two or more sequences in a row. End with Savasana.

► Add cardio to the mix: Do a 15-minute cardio workout of your choice before starting the yoga sequence.

► Add the Hilaria's Core Workout (page 236) in the middle of a sequence.

► Add five rounds of Sun Salutations (from the Yoga for Breathing sequence, page 68) into the middle of a sequence.

► Add extra restorative time at the end of any yoga practice; pull a blanket over your body, relax, get quiet, and rest in Savasana as long as you like.

My specific style of teaching is quite active, involving a lot of vinyasas—flowing sequences of one movement to another, coordinated to the breath. It's a bit like the Perfect Three in one exercise. The breath regulates the movement, with an inhale initiating an outward movement (a step, a stretch) and an exhale initiating a fold, a bend, or a release. The breath literally drives the movement of the body through space. In class, I talk students through a vinyasa by saying "inhale" and "exhale" on successive movements so they can truly drop into a flow without thinking about it.

So as you read the descriptions of each pose, please notice the breath instructions and inhale and exhale accordingly. The first time around, it may feel odd to read instructions for physical poses, but know that quickly they will sink into your muscle memory; after repeating a sequence a few times, you won't have to read, and the movements and breath work will feel natural.

TONING AND SCULPTING

Doing some kind of strength-building exercise is essential if you want to enjoy a body that is toned, nicely defined, and functions well in any activity. I've never met anyone who doesn't want to look good naked. If that's your goal, toning and sculpting have got to happen. Yoga on its own can often develop flexibility over strength, unless a teacher chooses to add pushups, core workouts, and other dynamic body-weight exercises into the practice. And it doesn't always offer the focused work on targeted muscles that contributes to sculpted legs, a toned derriere, and shoulders and arms you actually look forward to showing off.

There are many ways to work your muscles, and they bring different results.

Classic body-weight exercises—like pushups, squats, and lunges—can be done anytime (as part of cardio or yoga or on their own). Many of these are large, compound movements involving multiple muscle groups and joints—terrific not just for shaping your body but also for building the functional strength needed for everyday life, ensuring you don't injure yourself when picking up heavy bags and children. You might know many of these exercises from gym class already.

If you are able to train with supervision at a gym, you can learn how to use weights safely to load your body and maximize movements even more, which also builds bone

Classic Body-Weight Exercises You Can Do Anywhere

LOWER BODY

SQUATS AND VARIATIONS

WALL SITS

With your back pressed against the wall and your feet about 2 feet out from the wall, lower your butt until your thighs are parallel to the floor (as if seated on a chair). Make sure your knees are directly over your ankles and your shins are parallel to the wall. Engage your core and hold for 10 breaths.

LUNGES *(front, side, walking)*

CORE

HILARIA'S CORE WORKOUT *(page 236)*

PLANK AND VARIATIONS

SUPERMAN

Lying on your belly with your arms stretched out in front of you, activate your hamstrings, glutes, and lower back inhale lift your arms and legs at the same time, feeling your back body activate and lengthen and keeping your neck straight. Hold for 5 breaths.

UPPER BODY

PUSHUPS

PULLUPS

NEGATIVE PULLUPS *(easier for beginners)*

Holding an overhead bar, jump up to the top of a pullup position. Lower down super slow to a full hang. Repeat.

TRICEPS DIPS *(page 241)*

HILARIA'S CORE WORKOUT

This is the shortened version of the core sequence I teach in yoga class. If 10 repetitions are too hard, do 5.

1 DOLPHIN PLANK. Start in Plank with your feet together. Lower down onto your forearms, elbows directly underneath your shoulders, fingers outstretched, and palms planted firmly on the floor. Make sure your pelvis is parallel with the floor, engaging your core. Alternate leg lifts, doing 10 on each side. Push back through Child's Pose and into Boat Pose.

2 BOAT POSE. Balance on your sit bones, knees bent, holding your hands underneath your knees for support. Attempt to raise your feet a few inches above the ground and potentially let go of your knees. Breathe here or go further by bringing your shins and calves parallel with the floor, or go even further and extend your legs straight up, making a V shape with your body.

3 TWISTING BOAT POSE. With your legs off the floor and your knees bent if needed, sweep your arms over and to the right side, twisting your sternum. Sweep your arms over all the way left, twisting your sternum, feeling this in your obliques. Repeat five times on each side. Crunch all the way in, embracing your legs.

4 LEMON SQUEEZERS. Extend to a hover above the mat. Pulling your belly button toward your spine to engage your core, lift your chest and legs at the same time, toward each other, peeling your lower back off the floor and reaching your hands toward your toes, beyond your feet. Repeat 10 times. Release to the floor.

5 PILATES 100 PULSES + VARIATION. With your legs raised at a 45-degree angle and your knees bent if needed, actively reach your arms straight alongside your body. Lift your head and neck off your mat, and pulse your arms vigorously about 3 inches down and up. Repeat 20 times, inhaling for five pulses and exhaling for five. Maintain your leg position and hold the crunch at its peak. Encourage yourself to lift your torso just 1 inch higher, and then lower back down that same inch (no more!). Do 10 lifts. Repeat both exercises three times.

6 BICYCLE CRUNCHES. With your hands behind your head, draw your left knee to your belly button while lifting your chest up and twisting your right shoulder toward your left knee. Switch, keeping your elbows extremely wide and always fueling the movement from the center. Do 10 on each side. End facing forward with your knees and toes together and your legs still hovering off the floor.

7 CLAM CRUNCHES. Butterfly your knees open with your toes still together, keeping your hands behind your head and your elbows wide. Release your head and feet onto the floor, and then raise back up, crunching, your elbows and knees touching. Repeat 10 times. Repeat a second set. Release to the floor.

8 ROCK AND ROLL. Drawing your knees to your chest, wrap your arms around your knees, rock forward and back to build momentum, and come forward onto your hands and knees into Dolphin Plank.

9 In **DOLPHIN PLANK**, without moving your pelvis, bend your knees to almost touch the floor and then straighten them, keeping your pelvis parallel with the floor. Repeat 10 times.

10 SPHINX POSE. Lowering onto your belly, forearms pressing into the floor, move your elbows 1 inch forward with your fingers spread. Roll your shoulder blades down and back to lift your chest. Take five breaths. Release to the floor.

11 COBRA. Placing your hands on the floor on each side of your ribs, lift up into Low Cobra or High Cobra, maintaining your legs on the floor. Take five breaths.

density (critical to be aware of as we age). Done rapidly, this kind of strength training powerfully ups your heart rate and burns fat. Whether you're using machines or free weights or just doing drills in the park, the key with this kind of work is to focus and move rapidly from one movement to the next. (It's astonishing how many people stop between movements to text or check their e-mail!)

Barre workouts (also known as ballet barre) offer targeted fine-tuning work. Their small isometric movements—tensing the muscle while barely moving it—sculpt and carve the body beautifully over time but don't necessarily build functional strength. Many barre classes now combine both types of strength building in one—large and tiny movements—giving you the benefits of both. The key to maximizing barre class is to engage the core! All lower-body motion starts from here. Make sure to counter the "tightening" effect of barre class with good lower-body and shoulder stretches: Downward Facing Dog, Pigeon, Puppy, and Eagle Poses are your allies here.

> Apply the Five Principles and you will breathe through the hard parts, derive strength from grounded power, and benefit from core stability.

Body-weight workouts and barre classes are easy to find online. Many of the top barre studios, like Physique 57, stream classes to subscribers, and there are lots of free workouts online, as well. With any toning or strength work, it's paramount to put quality over quantity: Mastering the right form and only doing as many repetitions as you can while maintaining the right form will ensure you make gains rather than stress or strain yourself. A few minutes done well beats an hour done poorly. I recommend attending a class or gym-training session every so often to make sure your technique is on point.

Apply the Five Principles every time you tone, sculpt, and strengthen and you will breathe through the hard parts, derive strength from grounded power, and benefit from core stability. Each minute you do this, you are enhancing this incredible vehicle known as your body, revealing its full potential.

FOUND-MOMENTS EXERCISES

Becoming a mom meant that free time as I knew it before was gone, replaced by changing diapers, soothing to sleep, and making snacks. Often, grabbing 30 minutes in a row to do *anything* was literally impossible. So I did what all mothers do—stole 1 minute for myself here and 2 minutes there. I became a master multitasker, sneaking in butt-toning squeezes at the kitchen counter and crunches while Carmen did tummy time next to me on the rug, or jumping rope while doing the laundry. If I wanted to feel energized and limber, keep my mood up, and take good care of my body—especially after the amazing journey we'd been on, of pregnancy and birth—it had to happen in 1- or 2-minute intervals.

Astonishingly, the effects of these micro-workouts really did add up. When done with intention and awareness, they kept me lean, toned, and feeling good in my body. And they were like pressing the reset button on myself; if I felt dull, tired, or stiff, they quickly refreshed and relieved me.

The following little workout tricks can be the secret weapons in your exercise arsenal, whether you're time-challenged because of work, parenting, commuting, or all of the above. I use them constantly: scattered through busy workdays so I don't get sedentary, while traveling, or when watching my kids. By snacking on these healthy exercises throughout the day—think of them like the kale chips of exercise!—you stay in a good relationship with your body. You are always in a conversation, asking how it's feeling and keeping agile and strong. This can yield a bigger payback than ignoring it entirely until your one big workout of the day or week. Sure, you might look a little bit weird at times, but who wants to be normal? Normal is boring! And you might be surprised by who decides to follow along with you. Ultimately what works, wins.

Starting the Day

▸ After a morning shower, while your skin is air-drying, rev up your day with a quick set of barre exercises to work your butt and legs while standing at your sink with your feet parallel, hold on to the sink counter. Bend your left leg gently for support, extending your right leg behind you and bending your heel toward your butt. Poke your toe toward your butt 10 times, in tiny pulses. Keep your right knee aligned with your left. Flex your foot and do the same action for 10 presses. Point your toes again, maintaining the bent knee, and circle your leg first clockwise, then counterclockwise for 10 counts

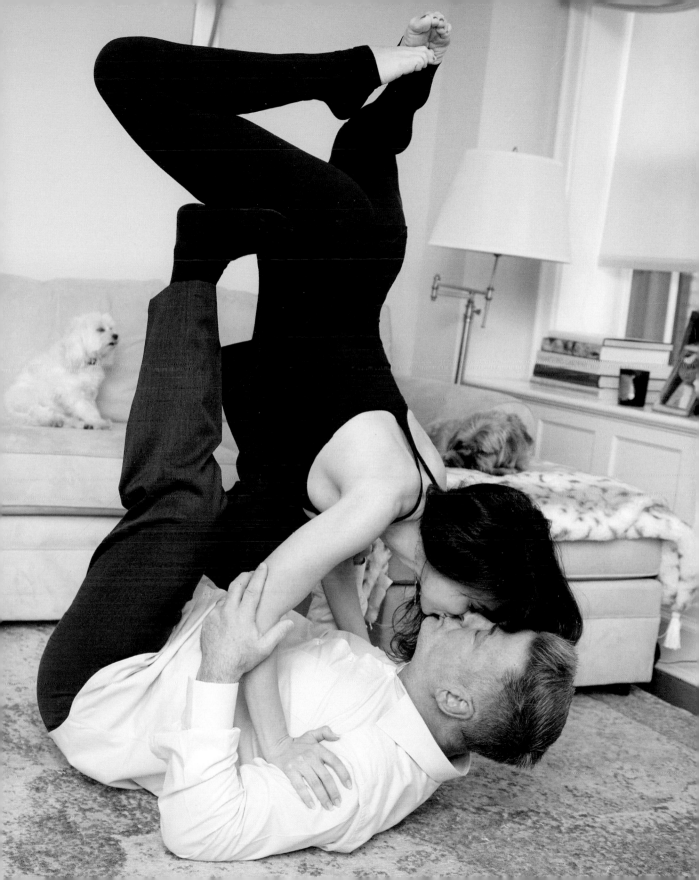

in each direction. Repeat on the other side and then do a standing Forward Fold for a counterstretch. Your hamstrings and glutes should be fired up!

► After putting on lotion, lie on a towel and do any of the exercises from Hilaria's Core Workout, or standard situps, before getting dressed.

Cleaning

► Do a Forward Fold while standing to activate your hamstrings and squats to strengthen your glutes while cleaning the bathroom and kitchen.

► While vacuuming, take a moment to stretch in the Pigeon Pose (page 126) and High Lunge (page 47).

► Use laundry time to go for a quick jog or toning session.

► Even ironing offers a moment to do Hamstring Curls: Bend your standing leg gently and extend the other leg straight behind you. Bend and straighten that leg, activating the hamstrings and glutes each time. Do 15 on each side.

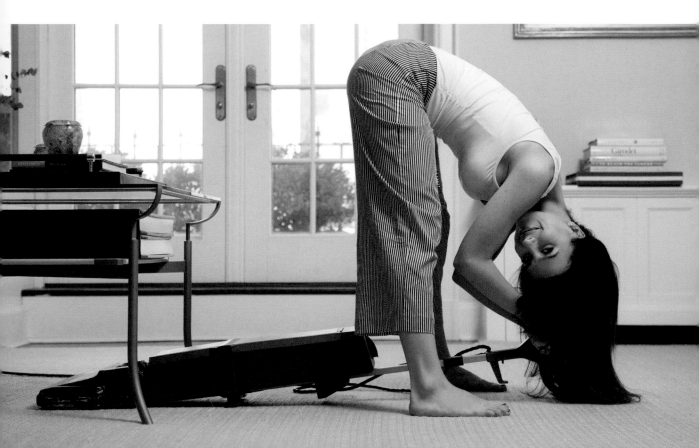

Watching TV

- Get on the floor and do Bridge Pose: Lie on your back, feet hip-distance apart and pressed firmly into the floor. Reach for your heels (you should be able to graze the backs of your feet with the tips of your fingers). Press into your heels and feet, and press your hips up into Bridge. Hold for five long breaths. Now lift your pelvis up and down to work your hamstrings and butt. Do 3 sets of 10.

- Do a core workout.

- Do Triceps Dips: Sit on your butt, with feet 1 foot in front, creating a V shape with the knees, and your arms behind you. Flex your feet. Lower and raise your body by bending your arms. Do 3 sets of 10.

Caring for Your Child

WITH A BABY

- Lie on your back, raise your knees to a crunch position, and play airplane: With your baby's tummy on your shins, hold her hips securely while flying her up and down, working your core.

- Crawl around with your baby, stopping to play Cat Cow and then raising your knees off the floor and holding Plank for strength.

- Playing peekaboo is a fun way to get in 10 squats while feeding your baby in a high chair; if you do jumps from a plié position, your baby will find it hilarious. This is also a great chance for Warrior 3 practice.

WITH A TODDLER

- Toddlers love to play alongside you as you do core work. Let your toddler count and you will both crack up.

- Teach your toddler a short yoga sequence. They are naturals at Downward Facing Dog and Cobra (and you'll reap the rewards if you teach your toddler Savasana).

- Practice Downward Facing Dog Split together, and then show her your one-legged pushups.

- Your toddler will love to climb on your back in Child's Pose and then hold on as you rise to all fours.

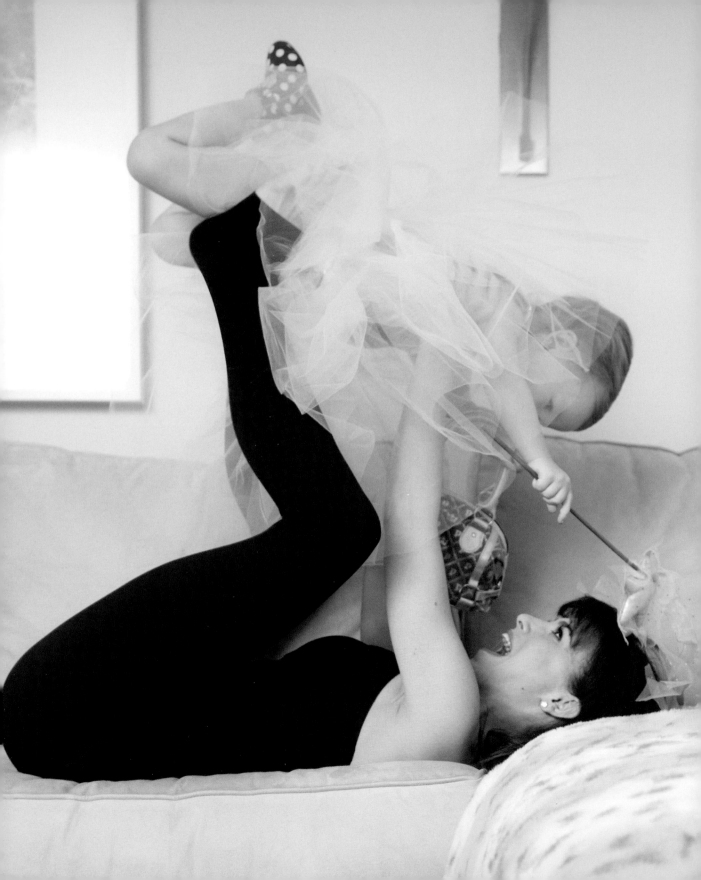

IN THE PARK AND PLAYGROUND

► Using your stroller handles for balance, hold a very wide second position until your inner thighs burn, and work the backs of your legs at stoplights by doing your morning barre exercises or Hamstring Curls. Or you can add something new: With your feet together, turn your toes out slightly, bend your standing leg, and lift your other leg up and back, keeping the turn out. Keep your leg straight and feel that your outer glutes and leg are activated. Pulse here for 15 counts. Repeat on the other side.

► With the feet in wide second position, sweep one arm overhead and into a deep side bend; switch sides. Do side bends, swooping your arm overhead.

► And don't just let your kid do all the running around; use playground time to work out. Run circles around your kid and do jumping jacks, squats, and jumping lunges (start in a high lunge and then jump, switching legs in midair; try doing 10) to get your cardio in. Use the steps and bars of the playground to do stepups (one leg at a time, moving slowly, pressing into your heel to work your glutes), pullups (even if you only get half an inch off the ground), and hanging leg lifts (hanging from an overhead bar, engage your core and pull your legs upward as far as you can, lower slowly, and repeat; bend your knees if needed). Keep your child in sight at all times—and don't get in any other kid's way if you want to stay friends with the other parents.

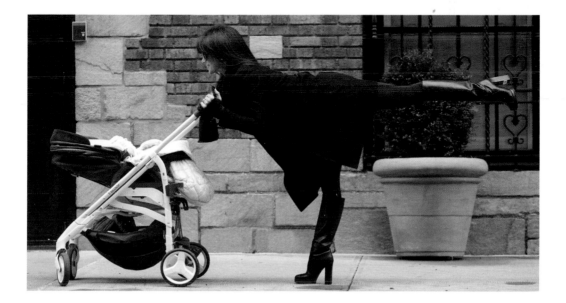

At Your Laptop

There are lots of ways to stay limber. Get off the chair and bring your laptop onto a flat surface.

▶ Alternate between Baddha Konasana and Wide Straddle (page 231) while reading or working. Baddha Konasana: Sit up tall (sit on a prop if this is too challenging), and butterfly your knees open, soles of your feet together. With your hands, draw your feet as close in toward your pelvis as possible and open your feet up to the ceiling like a little book. With a straight spine (no rounding!), bend forward for eight breaths.

▶ Take a brief break to stretch the front of your body and tone the back: Locust and Bow Poses. For Locust Pose, lie on your belly with your arms along your sides, pushing your belly into the floor. Raise your head, upper torso, arms, and legs off the floor on an inhale and hover on your belly and pelvis. Reach your arms back actively, keeping your gaze forward. Now bend your knees and bring your feet in toward your butt. Reach back to grab the tops of your feet (lasso them with a belt if you need help). Begin to kick up and back, pulling yourself into Bow Pose, continuously attempting to lift your knees off your mat, feeling an intense activation in your butt and a deep stretch through your chest and quads. Take five long breaths, release gently to the ground, and bring one cheek to the floor. From Locust's intense activation, now let go fully, softening and melting into the floor and allowing your hips to softly sway from side to side.

▶ Find a higher work surface, like a countertop, and alternate between sitting at your desk and standing to work during the day.

Standing Around

▶ With your feet hip-distance apart, do Relevé (page 90) with this variation: Tap your heels and squeeze your inner thighs, back to parallel, tap your heels and squeeze your inner thighs, back to parallel.

▶ A little ballet works well, too: Do Relevé 10 times, and then with your heels on the floor, turn your toes out and plié in first position, squeezing your thighs and activating your glutes as you lower and raise. Do this 10 times. Step your right foot back about 6 inches, keeping your toes turned out, into a ballet fourth position. With your right heel raised, bend and straighten your legs 10 times (curtsey plié). Switch legs.

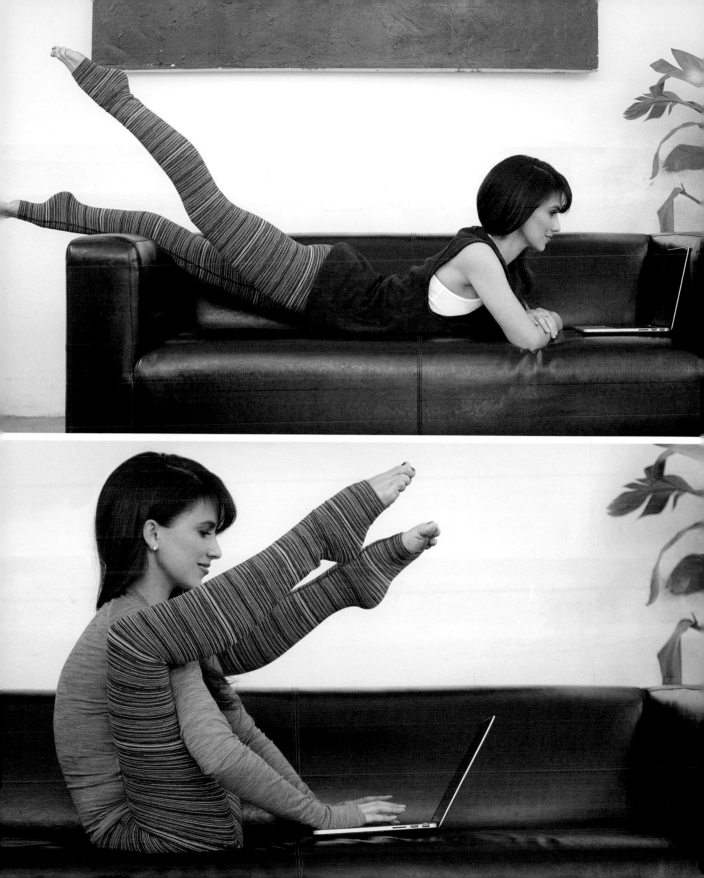

At Your Desk

- ► To relieve your upper back and shoulders, do Eagle Pose (page 231). As you type, periodically round and flex your back.

- ► Do inner-thigh squeezes as you sit and work to tone your legs.

- ► Put your legs up on each side of the computer to aid circulation. (*Warning:* This one is not skirt-friendly!)

- ► And the most powerful exercise of all: Get up from your desk every hour and move; doing some quick squats or jumping jacks is the fastest way to reboot energy and keep your lower body mobile.

Reading

▸ Do Wide-Leg Bridge Pose Lifts to work your butt and hamstrings. From Bridge Pose (page 241), release your pelvis down and step your feet about 5 inches away from your butt and widen them to the edges of your mat. Turn your toes out slightly and press into your heels as you flex your feet, lifting the pelvis up. Pulse or hold here.

▸ Do Frog Pose for a deep groin and inner-thigh stretch. Starting on the knees, split your knees wide, keeping your feet flexed, insteps on the floor, and heels wider than your knees, and release down onto your forearms. Keeping your pelvis in alignment with your knees, tuck your tailbone under, rounding your lower spine and activating your core. Press away with your forearms so your pelvis gently stretches toward your heels, feet still flexing. Breathe, holding the pose for 30 seconds to a couple of minutes. Do Low Lunge or Upward Dog afterward to open the hip flexors.

▸ Do Feet Up the Wall (page 102) for relaxing.

Ending the Day

To wind down before bed, turn all technology off and claim some "me" time. Do a quick core workout to fatigue your body nicely. Follow with: High Cobra, Child's Pose, Seated Forward Fold, and then lie on your back and pull one knee across your body in a twist. Follow with Happy Baby, Apanasana, and Savasana.

Cooking

While waiting for your water to boil or your baking to finish, use the kitchen counter to do some leg lifts, side bends, and calf raises or do drills running up and down stairs, squats, and jumping jacks.

Waiting for the Elevator

- Do Standing Half Hero's Pose (page 221).

- Do Bent-Knee Leg Raises: Standing on a gently bent left leg, raise your right knee to hip level. Tilt your torso slightly forward and engage your core. Lift your right knee 5 inches up, and then lower it to hip level. Repeat 10 times. Switch sides.

- Do Wall-Wide Pushups: Standing 2 feet away from the wall, place your hands on the wall wider than your shoulders. Engage your core tightly, and bring your torso and head toward the wall. Then push back slowly, keeping your body as straight as a plank the whole time. Repeat 10 times.

Grocery Shopping

Maximize that time strolling around the store by walking through the aisles on your tippy-toes—great for sculpting the legs. Activate your core!

Feeling Run Down

This is the time for quiet, restorative poses, like:

- Supta Baddha Konasana (page 127)

- Feet Up the Wall (page 102)

- Child's Pose and lots of Savasana

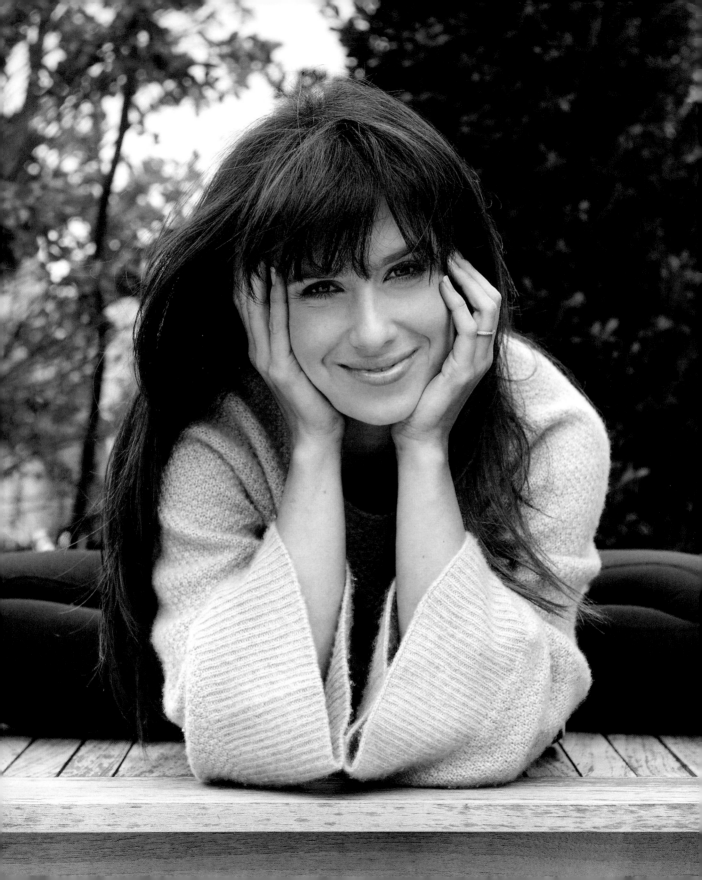

CONCLUSION

CONGRATULATIONS! WHILE YOU HAVE ARRIVED AT THE END OF THIS BOOK, understand that this is only just the beginning of your lifetime of Living Clearly. Remember, there is no one right way to use the information held in these pages. Living Clearly is not a precise science or a rigid step-by-step process, and it doesn't happen overnight. It is a practice that should be embraced playfully and integrated little by little into all the moments of your life. The yoga practices, exercises, recipes, and new ways of relating to people and situations can be customized to fit the unique shape and pace of your life. The only guideline that isn't optional is to commit to doing something from the book every day. Anything! Breaking old habits and forging a lasting new path is a gradual unfolding rather than a dramatic change. Do one positive thing for yourself each day and you'll find that the healthy energy builds upon itself. The more good things you do for yourself, the more good things you'll *want* to do for yourself. It can be as subtle as pausing before reacting, as significant as dropping a harmful addiction like smoking, or as simple as adding more movement (or vegetables) to your week.

Every moment is filled with possibilities. You can make a new dish for dinner, take a few minutes out of your day to explore a yoga pose, or practice a breathing exercise when you're stuck in traffic or pushed to your limit by your child or partner. Think of it as a series of experiments called "What will it feel like to make a different choice today?" Each time you choose something vibrant, energized, or positive, you make a deposit into your well-being bank account, investing in *you*. It starts to feel so good, it becomes increasingly harder to turn back.

In the beginning, it takes effort to choose something different, but even a step in a new direction builds momentum and develops muscle memory. It's like touch typing. When you are first learning to type, you painstakingly peck out your letters, but as your familiarity with the keyboard increases, you soon find yourself creating words, sentences, and even paragraphs without looking down—your fingers are flying, writing your thoughts, your hopes, your life. Your life is a book that *you* should author. This is how it works with wellness. Consciously feed yourself good food regularly, and your body will crave more of it. Stretch, run, and challenge your body regularly, and your muscles will ask you for more and more often—in an increasingly louder voice.

As you courageously dare yourself to make new choices along the road to Living Clearly, you'll never be alone on your journey. I'll be there with you. Turn to this book often, linger over a chapter or concept that speaks to you, or start over from the beginning again and again. The Living Clearly Method will lead you to more joy and fulfillment and an ever greater trust in your own capacity and greatness. Let this book be your trusty field guide along the way.

As you continue forward on your journey, remember that no one exactly like you has ever existed before, and no one will ever be quite like you again. Let your spirit shine so that when you look back, you simply have a collection of smiles, because you Lived Clearly, every single moment.

◂▲▸

ACKNOWLEDGMENTS

IN DEEP APPRECIATION, I THANK THE FOLLOWING PEOPLE, WHO HELPED TO bring this book to life.

Amely Greeven and Marisa Belger, not only for helping me refine my thousands of thoughts and ideas but also for being brilliant, strong mommies who brought so much wisdom into this book.

Melissa Petitto, my kitchen conspirator: You have taught me so much; you are my culinary soul mate.

Leah Miller, for taking an interest in my vision and life's work and giving me invaluable guidance. And the entire team at Rodale—I am so grateful and proud that I got to do this project with you, and I am thankful to call your publishing house my home.

Cait Hoyt, for believing in my philosophy and in me long before any spotlight had hit my name, and CAA for being a stellar team.

Jillian Taratunio and Yoel Najer, for making everything come together.

My family, students, friends, and teachers, who have seen me through my ups and downs and have inspired me to find happiness and create this method.

My babies, for bringing light and happiness into every day of my life.

And my husband, for being my *vida* and my *buen equipo*.

INDEX

Boldface page references indicate references indicate photographs. <u>Underscored</u> references indicate boxed text.